JUN 15 2004

D0198089

100 Questions & Answers About Bone Marrow and Stem Cell Transplantation

Ewa Carrier, MD
Gracy Ledingham

San Diego Public Library
LOGAN

JONES AND BARTLETT PUBLISHERS
Sudbury, Massachusetts
BOSTON TORONTO LONDON SINGAPORE

3 1336 06531 0071

JUN 1 5 2004

World Headquarters
Jones and Bartlett Publishers
40 Tall Pine Drive
Sudbury, MA 01776
info@jbpub.com
www.jbpub.com

Jones and Bartlett Publishers Canada
2406 Nikanna Road
Mississauga, ON L5C 2W6
CANADA

Jones and Bartlett Publishers International
Barb House, Barb Mews
London W6 7PA
UK

Copyright © 2004 by Jones and Bartlett Publishers, Inc.

All rights reserved. No part of the material protected by this copyright notice may be reproduced or utilized in any form, electronic or mechanical, including photocopying, recording, or by any information storage and retrieval system, without written permission from the copyright owner.

Library of Congress Cataloging-in-Publication Data

Carrier, Ewa.
100 questions & answers about bone marrow and stem cell transplantation / Ewa Carrier, Gracy Ledingham.
p. cm.
Includes bibliographical references and index.
ISBN 0-7637-1273-6
1. Bone marrow--Transplantation--Miscellanea. 2. Bone marrow--Transplantation--Popular works. 3. Hematopoietic stem cells--Transplantation--Miscellanea. 4. Hematopoietic stem cells--Transplantation--Popular works. I. Title: One hundred questions and answers about bone marrow and stem cell transplantation. II. Ledingham, Gracy. III. Title.
RD123.5.C37 2003
617.4'4--dc21

200300846

The authors, editors, and publisher have made every effort to provide accurate information. However, they are not responsible for errors, omissions, or for any outcomes related to the use of the contents of this book and take no responsibility for the use of any products described herein. Treatments and side effects described in this book may not be applicable to all patients; likewise, some patients may require a dose or experience a side effect that is not described herein. The reader should confer with his or her own physician regarding specific treatments and side effects. Drugs and medical devices are discussed that may have limited availability or be controlled by the Food and Drug Administration (FDA) for use only in a research study or clinical trial. The drug information presented has been derived from reference sources, recently published data, and pharmaceutical research data. Research, clinical practice, and government regulations often change the accepted standard in this field. When consideration is being given to use of any drug in the clinical setting, the health care provider or reader is responsible for determining FDA status of the drug, reading the package insert, reviewing prescribing information for the most up-to-date recommendations on dose, precautions, and contraindications, and determining the appropriate usage for the product. This is especially important in the case of drugs that are new or seldom used. Comments from a patient or patients used in this text are the opinions of the commenter and should not be construed as representative of the authors' or publisher's viewpoint.

Production Credits:
Acquisitions Editor: Christopher Davis
Production Editor: Elizabeth Platt
Cover Design: Philip Regan
Manufacturing Buyer: Therese Bräuer
Composition: Northeast Compositors
Printing and Binding: Malloy Lithographing
Cover Printer: Malloy Lithographing

Printed in the United States of America
07 06 05 04 03 10 9 8 7 6 5 4 3 2 1

Contents

Foreword

Gracy Ledingham, BMT Patient
November, 2002

One afternoon we were trimming the rubber tree in our backyard. When we finished, I noticed that there were bruises on my arms. The next day the bruises were still there. The bruises were not healing because I had developed leukemia. Doctors would call it a very aggressive form of leukemia. When doctors talk about "aggressive form," think, "why am I still alive?" At that point we boarded a roller coaster for a ride that lasted two years and continues today. We've taken in all the sights, from chemotherapy to irradiation and, finally, bone marrow transplantation (BMT). The bone marrow transplant is what this book is about, but the story is also about my journey.

At the beginning my husband and I had many questions. Getting them answered was tiring and frustrating in itself. The scientific information was hard to interpret. Descriptions of the disease on the Internet go into great detail but provided little that was helpful to us on the personal coping level. Other cancer patients, while good for support and full of cancer information, knew little of the BMT process. Doctors and nurses tried to be helpful, but we had so many questions about practical things and their focus was on the disease itself. We think that hearing about the BMT from someone who went through it might be helpful to others.

We hope the toughest part of this trip is over. Of course, with cancer there are no long-term promises. We now know many of the answers to those questions we had before going through this. We are still learning the answers to new questions as we move along. Most importantly, we've learned that there are some questions for which there are no answers. We hope this book will answer some of your questions and perhaps help you to ask some of your own.

If you are browsing through this book because you or someone you love is about to go through the bone marrow transplant process, there is something very important you should know. This experience is going to be a transforming event in your life and the lives of all who love you. We are not talking about the medical procedure. You are going to come out on the other side of this a different person than you were when you went in. This is going to happen whether you want it to or not. It is also going to change those who love you. Whether the new person is better than the old one is going to be completely up to you. This is a chance to learn about yourself, those you love, and life.

Although it may be hard to believe at this point in your life, this is an opportunity. As we look back today, both of us—Gracy and John (Gracy's partner in life)—know that who we are today is much more than who we were before the bone marrow transplant.

Introduction

Patients who are eligible for stem cell transplant usually are those who have undergone chemotherapy that didn't work or who have disease with a very high risk of rapid decline and death. Very frequently, they have been told that unless they go through stem cell transplant, they will die within weeks or months. Stem cell transplant is therefore a last-chance, life-saving procedure for them. They face death unless they subject themselves to transplant. For me, it is a situation that requires significant focus and effort. Any decision made lightly could make a difference between life and death. If a patient dies, I accept it in my heart, but when a patient survives, I celebrate and plant a rose in my garden. Each survival is a gift that I hold and treasure and gain strength from.

The transplant procedure has a tremendous emotional charge. Patients are scared and intimidated. However, there is something beyond their physical body that supports them, which is their mental and spiritual strength. If this strength is enhanced, they frequently make it against all odds. If this strength is suppressed, they fall apart. I believe that physicians and supporting staff must go beyond the routine to see the person behind the procedure—to enhance this invisible quality and let it shine.

My coauthor and patient, Gracy Ledingham, had a very serious, high-risk leukemia. Her white cell count was 400,000 compared to a count of 4,000 for a healthy individual. She also had a genetic mutation called 4/11 translocation, biphenotypic type, that indicates an extremely high-risk illness. When told how dangerous her condition could be and that transplant was the only option, she embraced the news with courage, strength, and, yes, grace, and prepared herself for the procedure. Her sister flew in from Taiwan, and Gracy received 6/6 allogeneic stem cell transplant. Throughout the procedure she was strong, informed, and ahead of the game. She took notes and always asked questions. She empowered herself with knowledge and vision. Now, three years post transplant, she is leukemia free, off medications, and has a new outlook on life, which she will project in this book.

We would like this book to be a source of information for frightened patients awaiting stem cell transplant. A source of encouragement and strength. A guide in days ahead.

Performing stem cell transplants gives me joy and a deep sense of fulfillment. I consider it a privilege to work with people who face such tremendous adversity, and I admire them for their courage, perseverance, and optimism. I learn from them every day.

I could not do this work without my children, Nathalie and Matt, whose support and patience is beyond limitations. I am grateful to my mother, who taught me how to love life and people, and I thank my patients—Krystal, Gracy, Monica, Karen, Emmit, Simon, Joseph, and many others—for their courage and example. Finally, I would like to thank my boss and mentor, Dr. Edward Ball, for his quiet and consistent encouragement, inspiration, and support. He created an environment in which performing these transplants is a daily source of satisfaction.

Ewa Carrier, MD

PART ONE

The Basics

What is bone marrow? Why might someone need a bone marrow transplant?

What is a stem cell?

How was BMT discovered as a treatment for blood diseases?

More . . .

1. What is bone marrow? Why might someone need a bone marrow transplant?

Bone marrow
the soft, fatty substance filling the cavities of the bones where blood cells are made.

Cell
the basic structural unit of all life. All living matter is composed of at least one cell.

Peripheral blood
blood that passes through the arteries and veins to supply oxygen to the tissues and organs.

Immune system
a complex system by which the body protects itself from harmful foreign substances and organisms.

Leukemia
a malignancy of a white blood cell in which there is an accumulation of abnormal white blood cells in the blood and the bone marrow.

Leukocyte
a white blood cell or corpuscle.

Bone marrow is a spongy tissue inside the bones that produces blood (Figure 1). All blood **cells** develop from immature cells called hematopoietic (blood-forming) stem cells (see Question 2). Most of the stem cells that can form blood are found in the bone marrow, but some may circulate in the **peripheral blood**—that is, the blood that passes through your arteries and veins to supply oxygen to your tissues and organs.

When a person develops or is born with a disease of the bone marrow or the blood, such as leukemia, sickle cell anemia, and similar disorders, it means that some of the person's blood cells do not function properly. Poorly functioning blood cells can affect not only the ability of blood to bring oxygen and nutrients to bodily tissues, but also can prevent the **immune system** from functioning properly. In the case of some cancers, the bone marrow may also be producing too many of these malfunctioning cells. In **leukemia**, for example, blood cells called **leukocytes**—cells that, when they function properly, fight infections—fail to develop normally. These cells are also produced more quickly than normal and crowd out healthy leukocytes. The abnormal cells cannot fight infections, so the person with leukemia is vulnerable to life-threatening illnesses such as pneumonia and sepsis. That is why it is essential to "re-set" a person's bone marrow to start making healthy cells again. One way to do this is to add healthy hematopoietic stem cells into the body in the hope that these stem cells will take over the job of producing healthy cells in the bone marrow.

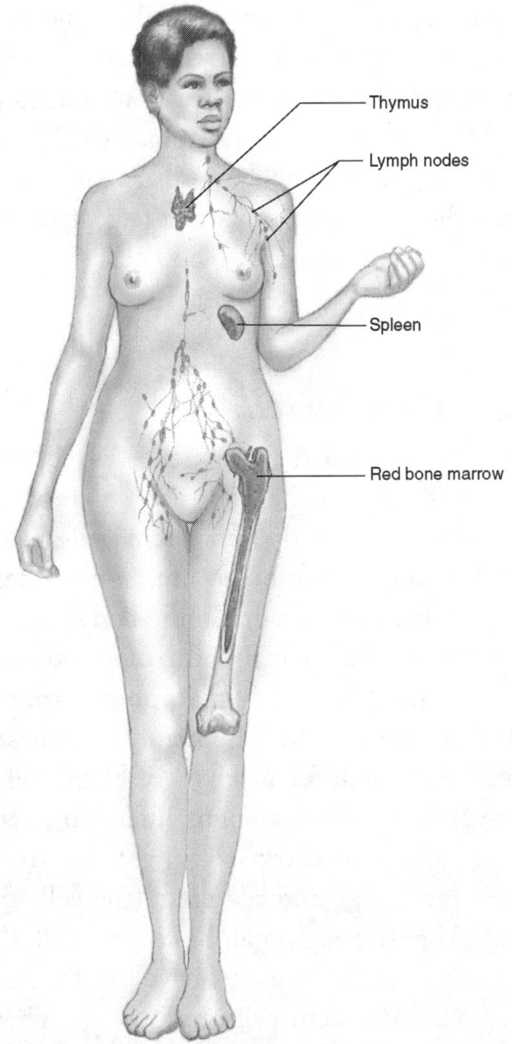

Figure 1 The immune system. Many of the diseases treated with BMT and SCT, such as leukemia, lymphoma, and systemic lupus erythematosus, are disorders of the immune system. The white blood cells that are the foundation of the immune system are formed in the bone marrow and "trained" to recognize invading cells by the thymus gland. These cells circulate through the body via lymphatic vessels, lymph nodes, and the spleen as well as through blood vessels (not shown). In cancers of the blood, such as leukemia or lymphoma, the bone marrow produces large numbers of white blood cells that are not fully formed and cannot fight disease; transplantation is intended to halt this overproduction. In other blood diseases, such as systemic lupus erythematosus, the cells overreact and attack normal, healthy cells in the body, so transplanted cells are intended to bring down the level of immune response.

The stem cells may be taken from the bone marrow or the blood (see Question 3) and therefore the terms used for the transplant procedure are **bone marrow transplant** (BMT) or **stem cell transplant** (SCT). The different names simply refer to different methods of achieving the same goal: obtaining new stem cells for a person whose own source of blood cells does not work properly.

Bone marrow transplant (BMT)
transplantation of stem cells collected from bone marrow.

Stem cell transplant
the process by which new stem cells are infused into a patient.

Stem cell
a primitive type of cell from which all cells of a given organ or tissue arise.

Hematopoietic stem cell transplant
the process by which new stem cells are introduced into a patient.

White blood cell
a blood cell that does not contain hemoglobin; also called leukocyte.

Red blood cells
hemoglobin-containing blood cells that carry oxygen to the tissues.

Platelet
a cell formed by the bone marrow and circulating in the blood that is necessary for blood clotting.

2. What is a stem cell?

A **stem cell** is a cell that can renew itself and make other types of cell in the body. There are three basic types of stem cells: totipotent stem cells, which can restore all tissues in the body; multipotent stem cells, which can form many tissues in the body; and mulipotent stem cells, which can form many kinds of the same tissue, including the **hematopoietic stem cell**, or the cell that forms blood. The hematopoietic stem cell can form all three different kinds of blood cells: **white blood cells** (the cells that fight infection), **red blood cells** (the cells that carry oxygen to the tissues and organs of the body), and **platelets** (the cells that heal wounds). Almost every organ has a stem cell: the brain has neural stem cells, muscles have muscle stem cells, the liver has liver stem cells, and so on. These stem cells live in the organ in a dormant state and may multiply and differentiate when tissue damage occurs. The hematopoietic stem cells respond to a signal that there is not enough blood in the person's circulatory system and will form white blood cells, red blood cells, or platelets as needed. Researchers recently have learned that hematopoietic stem cells can form other types of cells, such as liver cells and muscle cells. This ability of stem cells to change from one tissue to another tissue is called "stem cell plasticity."

3. How was BMT discovered as a treatment for blood diseases?

BMTs done in the late 1950s to the late 1960s were often disappointing. Most patients who had transplants were terminally ill and often died soon after the transplant. Many patients receiving BMT were given bone marrow that was not typed correctly. Some patients died of **graft-versus-host disease (GVHD),** in which the transplanted tissue attacks the person it was supposed to cure, or succumbed to infections that took advantage of the patient's weakened immune system.

Graft-versus-host disease (GVHD)
a situation in which the lymphocytes from a donor's stem cells recognize certain antigens on the recipient (patient) as foreign.

HLA typing
tests to determine the antigens present in a person's cells.

In the early 1970s there were dramatic improvements in the survival rates of patients undergoing the procedure. This was due to **HLA typing**, which was established around that time (see Question 14). BMTs were also more successful because leukemia patients received transplants while in **remission** and because supportive care had improved. The results of BMTs continued to improve through the 1970s and 1980s as new antibacterial, antifungal, and antiviral agents were developed. At the same time, medications called **growth factors** were developed, which increased the patients' neutrophil counts so they had fewer infections. Today, the cure rate for acute leukemia patients receiving BMT is about 50–70%; for chronic myelogenous leukemia, it's about 70–80%; and for aplastic anemia, it's 60–80%. In the relatively short time of about four decades, the bone marrow transplant procedure has become a successful form of treatment for a number of illnesses. Many patients who would die otherwise can be saved through the BMT. The use of blood as a stem cell source redefined this procedure to stem cell transplant (SCT), but

Remission
complete or partial disappearance of the signs and symptoms of disease in response to treatment; the period during which a disease is under control.

Growth factors
proteins that encourage blood cells to reproduce more rapidly. These are generally used to restore white blood cell counts following treatment.

Many patients who would die otherwise can be saved through the BMT.

the basic idea is the same: stem cells from a healthy **donor** are used to replace diseased tissue.

Donor
a healthy person who donates blood stem cells or bone marrow for infusion into a patient.

4. What is the difference between BMT and SCT?

When doctors first developed procedures for transplanting stem cells, they were performing only the bone marrow transplant procedure at first—stem cells could only be taken directly from bone marrow. Doctors performed the **bone marrow harvest** in the operating room while the donor was under under general anesthesia. The donor's marrow was **aspirated** with a special needle. Then, doctors filtered the harvested cells and infused them into the blood stream of the patient (just like a blood transfusion). Usually, the donor could go home after the harvest procedure and just take Tylenol for pain. This procedure did not have negative **side effects**, but required the patient to be admitted to a surgery unit and have general anesthesia.

Bone marrow harvest
collection of stem cells from marrow for later infusion into the patient.

Aspirate
removing fluid or cells by inserting a needle into tissue and drawing the fluid into the syringe.

Side effects
effects of treatment other than the desired effects.

Since then, however, scientists have learned more about stem cell transplantation, and doctors now use a substance called **granulocyte-colony stimulating factor** (G-CSF) or **granulocyte macrophage-colony stimulating factor** (GM-CSF) to move stem cells out of the donor's bone marrow into the peripheral blood, where the cells can be retrieved from the blood by a process called apheresis (see Question 36). This procedure is easier on the donors because they do not have to be admitted into a hospital, they do not need general anesthesia, and they usually do not feel pain afterwards.

Granulocyte-colony stimulating factor (G-CSF)
a growth factor (protein) given to activate production of cells. A second factor, granulocyte macrophage-colony stimulating factor (GM-CSF), may also serve the same purpose.

5. *What kinds of transplants can be performed?*

There are several kinds of transplants: **autologous**, **allogeneic**, and **syngeneic**. The choice of transplant depends on the disease, the patient's condition, and in some cases the availability of a donor. Allogeneic transplants use cells from another person. Autologous transplants use the patient's own healthy stem cells. Syngeneic transplants use cells from the patient's identical twin, so it is less commonly performed, but when an identical twin donor is available, the results are better than when the donor is unrelated. If a patient isn't lucky enough to have an identical twin (most don't), a sibling is usually the best alternative. Matched sibling transplant is associated with fewer complications and side effects than when the donor is not related to the patient. The one exception to this general rule is when **cord blood** is used to transplant stem cells in children (see Question 15); even when the cord blood is from someone not related to the child needing the transplant, there are few side effects.

Autologous transplantation
transplantation using stem cells from the patient's own body.

Allogeneic stem cell transplantation
transplant procedure using cells from another person to treat a cancer.

Syngeneic transplant
a stem cell transplant from an identical twin.

Doctors perform autologous transplants, which use a patient's own marrow, for diseases such as multiple myeloma, lymphoma, solid tumors, and autoimmune disorders (lupus erythematosus, multiple sclerosis, Crohn's disease, rheumatoid arthritis, etc.). Allogeneic and unrelated transplants are used for younger patients with high-risk leukemia and lymphomas. Thus, allogeneic and unrelated transplants are usually limited to younger patients with high-risk diseases because these transplants are very risky. Patients need high-dose chemotherapy and frequently radiation therapy to suppress the immune system (see Question 14), which puts them at risk for serious, even life-threatening, infections. Because another person's cells are introduced into the body, there is also a risk that the new cells will attack the patient's own cells, a condition called graft-versus-host disease (GVHD). Thus, allogeneic transplants are used only when absolutely necessary for patients who can expect to live a long time if the transplant is successful.

Allogeneic transplants are only used when absolutely necessary.

6. Which of the different types of transplant require a stay in a bone marrow transplant unit?

Allogeneic stem cell transplant is a high-risk procedure that must be performed in a BMT unit. This unit is a specialized area of the hospital with a special filtration system that decreases microbial agents in the air. The unit is staffed by experienced nurses, nurse practitioners, and case managers so that critically ill patients can be well tended. The unit is usually located close to the Intensive Care Unit so that patients whose condition worsens can be transferred there quickly. The BMT unit should be located in an area that has low staff and visitor traffic; it is very dangerous to expose BMT patients to people who may carry infections, so contact with people must be minimized.

Although allogeneic transplants must be performed in a BMT unit, there is another form of allogeneic transplant, called a "mini-allogeneic" transplant, that is less risky and has fewer side effects (see Question 16). Also, autologous transplants—those using the patient's own stem cells—are less invasive and may be performed in the regular Hematology/Oncology Unit or even on an outpatient basis.

7. *What happens in stem cell transplantation?*

Stem cell transplantation has two steps. First, the patient will be given **chemotherapy** and/or **radiation therapy** to suppress the immune system, kill any remaining cancer cells or auto-sensitized cells, and create a space in the bone marrow. The patient receives chemotherapy over several days, and in most cases it is well tolerated. The patient may have radiation therapy before or after chemotherapy, several times a day. A radiation oncologist will decide on the dose and frequency of irradiation. **Hyperfractionation** or **fractionated treatment**—small doses of radiation given in several sessions—is designed to reduce side effects and limit damage to healthy tissues. The patient receives **total body irradiation** (TBI) to suppress the patient's immune system and prevent rejection of the incoming cells (see Questions 71–74). The procedure itself is painless but may cause nausea and a decrease in energy. Patients can take medications to control nausea and vomiting. In the case of mini-allogeneic transplants or nonmyeloablative stem cell transplants (see Question 16), the radiation dose (if any) is very small and should not cause any side effects. After a day of rest, stem cells are infused into the patient's bloodstream in a manner similar to a blood transfusion, usually over the period of 1 to 2 hours. The recovery time is about 2 weeks for autologous transplant and 4 weeks for allogeneic transplant. Infused cells circulate in the blood for several days before they find their way into the bone marrow cavity and begin to grow. This process is called homing. During stem cell recovery, the patient is **immunocompromised**—that is, his or her immune system is

Chemotherapy
treatment of cancer by use of chemicals, and often uses two or more chemicals to achieve maximum kill of tumor cells. Usually refers to drugs used to treat cancer.

Radiation therapy
treatment with high energy x-rays to destroy cancer cells and suppress the immune system.

Hyperfractionation
a dose of radiation given in several sessions instead of all at once. Also called fractionated treatment.

Total body irradiation (TBI)
radiation therapy given over the whole body to remove all cancer or disease cells and suppress the immune system.

Immunocompromised
a condition in which a patient's immune system is unable to perform its functions adequately, leaving the patient vulnerable to infections.

unable to perform adequately, so he or she is vulnerable to infections. For this reason, the patient needs to remain in a room with special ventilation systems and take antibiotics to prevent infections.

8. Who requires stem cell transplantation? How is this decision made?

There are a number of diseases that can be treated with BMT or SCT. Table 1 lists the diseases for which transplant is effective. Most patients are referred for transplant after other therapies have failed.

The transplant procedure is complicated and requires patient and doctor cooperation.

The goal of the transplant is cure. From the point of view of both the patient and the transplant unit, deciding to go forward with the transplant procedure is complicated and requires patient and doctor cooperation. Underlying disease, the extent of previous chemotherapy, the availability of a donor (for allogeneic transplant), and the availability of social and family support are all factors in this decision. Many transplant centers conduct a new patient conference weekly to discuss each new patient's eligibility for transplant. All doctors, nurses, case managers, and a social worker are present and voice their opinions. They extensively discuss the benefits and the possible dangers for each patient—a necessity, as all patients' circumstances are different, and no one wants to give a treatment to a patient who will not benefit from it (and might even suffer further harm).

9. What is outpatient transplant?

Recent improvement in supportive care and changes in the economy have forced many transplant centers to perform autologous and "mini-allogeneic" stem cell transplants (see Question 16) on an outpatient basis.

Table 1 Diseases treated with bone marrow or stem cell transplant

Diseases treated with bone marrow or stem cell transplant
Aplastic anemia
Acute lymphoblastic leukemia (ALL)
Acute myelogenous leukemia (AML)
Beta-thalassemia
Crohn's disease (experimental)
Chronic myelogenous leukemia (CML)
Fanconi's anemia
Hodgkin's disease (HD)
Multiple myeloma (MM)
Multiple sclerosis (MS)
Myelodysplastic syndrome (MDS)
Non-Hodgkin's lymphoma (NHL)
Renal carcinoma
Sarcomas
Severe combined immunodeficiency disease (SCID)
Sickle cell disease (SCD)
Systemic lupus erythematosus (SLE)
Wiskott-Aldrich Syndrome

Patients may stay in a hotel room or at home and can be checked daily at an infusion center. This approach has significantly lowered the cost of transplant without compromising the quality of patient care. In order to receive an outpatient transplant, the patient must be compliant and have a reliable caregiver who can accompany the patient to and from the hospital at all times. The patient must also undergo a **conditioning regimen** and, if he or she does not already live near the transplant center, a temporary home or hotel room near such a center is required. Such centers are becoming common in many areas of the country, which in turn increases the availability of mini-allogeneic transplants. Full allogeneic transplants, however, must be performed on an in-patient basis.

Conditioning regimen
chemotherapy designed to prepare for transplant by suppressing the immune system and killing cancer cells.

10. How long after the diagnosis should the transplant take place?

The timing of your transplant will depend on your disease.

The timing of your transplant will depend on your disease. Some patients can (and should) have a transplant immediately; for example, younger patients with acute myelogenous leukemia who have poor **risk factors** and a matched sibling donor may be encouraged to have a transplant soon after the diagnosis, although it is best to do this after **induction therapy**. Induction therapy is given shortly after the diagnosis to decrease the **bulk** (amount) of the disease. In the case of chronic myelogenous leukemia (CML), the patient may be prescribed standard chemotherapy agents or a new drug called Gleevec, which is very effective for CML; if these do not work, transplantation is the next step. Multiple myeloma is also treated with transplantation early because this disease can return even after a successful round of chemotherapy; the transplant helps to prolong disease-free survival.

Risk factors
anything that increases an individual's chance of getting a disease such as cancer.

Induction therapy
chemotherapy that suppresses the patient's immune system prior to transplantation.

Bulk
amount of disease.

In some other cases, however, there are good reasons to wait. There are many risks with BMT and SCT, so patients who have just been diagnosed and who have few serious risk factors generally have chemotherapy first, with transplantation the "last resort." For example, in patients with acute lymphoblastic leukemia (ALL), risk factors determine whether the transplant is considered early in therapy. If the patient has no serious risk factors, such as high initial white cell count or specific genetic translocations (see Question 42), he or she receives standard chemotherapy. If the leukemia resists standard treatment or the patient **relapses**, then early transplant is considered.

Relapse
the reappearance of cancer after a disease-free period.

Even when it's clear that the patient needs a transplant, some diseases, such as non-Hodgkin's lymphoma, must be treated with **consolidation chemotherapy** first to get the patient into complete or partial remission. This can take some time. Also, if it's possible for the patient to have time to recover from previous chemotherapy before the transplant, it is a good idea to do so—a patient weakened from chemotherapy will suffer less from the transplant if he or she has a chance to recover. If the disease is not immediately life-threatening, doctors generally choose this option. It is important in these cases for the doctor to carefully monitor the patient's condition to make sure that waiting is not going to be harmful in the long run.

Consolidation chemotherapy
additional chemotherapy given after induction chemotherapy.

11. What is the success rate of stem cell transplant?

The success rate depends on the type of disease, the age of the patient, the type of transplant, and the extent of previous chemotherapy. For CML, when the optimal donor is available the success rate can be close to 75%. For acute leukemias, the success rate may be close to 50–60%. In lymphomas, the results depend on the stage and status of the disease at the time of the transplant. In most cases, 50% of the patients are expected to be alive after five years. In systemic lupus erythematosus (SLE) and multiple sclerosis (MS), for which transplantation is still experimental, most patients will benefit from transplant, but we still don't know how long the remission will last.

In most lymphoma cases, 50% of the patients are expected to be alive after five years.

AUTOLOGOUS TRANSPLANTS

12. When is autologous transplant performed?

Autologous transplant is performed when the patient's own healthy bone marrow or peripheral blood stem cells can be used. These healthy cells are extracted from the patient, frozen, and stored for later use. Chemotherapy and, rarely, radiation therapy are then given to the patient to destroy cancerous cells. This treatment also destroys bone marrow and makes space for the stem cells that will be infused. The stored stem cells are then re-infused into the patient to restore the function of his or her bone marrow and shorten the period of **neutropenia** (low white blood cell count). Usually, autologous transplants are done when the bone marrow is healthy and the disease is somewhere else in the body. Sometimes, however, autologous transplant is done in patients with multiple myeloma and leukemia, illnesses in which the bone marrow itself is diseased. In these cases, the bone marrow may be **purged** before infusion, that is, cleansed of the cancerous cells, so that only healthy cells remain.

Neutropenia

a condition wherein the body is depleted of important disease-fighting white blood cells.

Purge

to clean out or remove diseased cells from tissue, in this case bone marrow.

13. Can autologous stem cells be completely purged of cancer cells?

When stem cells are collected from the patient for autologous transplant, it's always possible that cancer cells can contaminate the stem cells. To lessen this risk, stem cells are usually collected from patients while they are in remission—that is, at times when their disease appears to be inactive, and their blood cells are being produced and are functioning normally. Unfortunately, even when a patient is in remission, tumor cells sometimes can be hiding in apparently normal marrow or blood products used for transplantation, and these hidden cells may contribute to a relapse. There are several methods used to purge stem cells of cancer cells before transplant, but we don't know if any of these methods can remove *all* of the cancer cells. To determine with any degree of certainty which methods work best, we would have to perform large-scale clinical studies comparing the various purging techniques—studies that would require a large number of patients to participate to be worthwhile. No such studies have been performed to date. So at this point, the answer to the question is simply that there's no way to be sure, and autologous transplantation is therefore a calculated risk.

ALLOGENEIC TRANSPLANTS

14. How is a suitable donor identified for allogeneic transplants?

Allogeneic transplant is performed in younger patients with aggressive disease, such as high-risk leukemias and lymphomas. To find a donor, the patient and the donor need to be tested for the compatibility of their **human leukocyte antigens (HLA)**. These antigens are a kind of "fingerprint" for one's own cells, and they play an important role in the body's ability to distinguish between "self" and the "other." If your antigens match the donor's antigens, there is a good chance that stem cells from the donor will be accepted by and grow in your body. If the antigens do not match, the reaction called graft-versus-host disease (GVHD) may occur, or there may be a **graft failure** (see Question 75).

Human leukocyte antigen (HLA)
antigens that act as markers on each person's cells that help the body distinguish its own cells from invading or foreign cells.

When the stem cells come from a relative, usually a sibling, in whom all 6 of the 6 HLA antigens are identical to the patient's HLA antigens (referred to as a 6/6 match), the transplant is called a **matched sibling transplant (MST)**. If the stem cells are obtained from an unrelated donor, the transplant is called a **matched unrelated donor (MUD) transplant**.

Matched sibling transplant (MST)
a transplant in which the stem cells come from a relative, usually a sibling, in whom all 6 of the 6 HLA antigens are identical to the patient's HLA antigens.

Matched unrelated donor (MUD) transplant
a transplant in which the stem cells are obtained from an unrelated donor whose HLA antigens match at least some of the patient's.

15. What is a cord blood transplant?

Cord blood is blood collected from a baby's placenta and umbilical cord at the time of birth. Although it is not yet common for people to preserve this blood, more parents are choosing to do so because scientists have discovered that the blood in the umbilical cord has many stem cells that can be transplanted later.

Several hundred cord blood transplants have been performed to date, and the data suggest that these transplants may have a lower risk of GVHD. Cord blood can be collected from both the umbilical cord and the placenta after birth. If the umbilical cord is clamped within 30 seconds of vaginal delivery while the placenta is still inside the mother, an experienced physician can collect up to 100 milliliters of cord blood without harming either the infant or the mother. Cord blood is generally not manipulated before it is frozen and stored, so the stem cells can be preserved.

Considering the advantages of cord blood transplants—lower risk of GVHD for the recipient and completely painless collection for the donor infant—it seems strange that so few have been performed, until you understand the reasons why doctors are *not* collecting cord blood. Congenital malformations in the child are one rationale—and a sensible one, considering that no one knows how the genetic problems of the donor child might affect the already sick recipient. Cord blood banks test all collected cord blood for infections and for possible congenital malformations. But the other primary reason is simply that the mother has not given her informed consent for the procedure. However, as more people become aware of the possibilities of cord blood transplants, preserving cord blood is becoming more common. However, the number of stem cells obtained from one newborn baby is relatively small and usually not enough to successfully transplant an adult patient. Most cord blood transplants have been performed in children.

With cord blood collected for an unrelated transplant, doctors study the medical histories of both the biological mother and father. Also, before the cells may be used for transplant, the donor infant must be evaluated at 6 and 12 months of age for any evidence of congenital or infectious diseases that might not have been obvious at birth. Cord blood contamination (inadvertent contamination with bacteria or other infectious agents during the collection procedure) rates are reported to be 3–15%. This depends on what kind of collection system was used. The possibility of contamination means that the cord blood must undergo stringent microbiological testing before it is used.

Nonmyeloablative stem cell transplant (NST)

an allogeneic transplant with less toxicity in which only part of the patient's bone marrow is destroyed by chemotherapy before the transplant.

Chimerism

the presence of both patient and donor cells together in the bone marrow. Full donor chimera transformation of a patient's bone marrow to match the bone marrow of his or her donor.

16. What is the "mini-allogeneic" transplant?

This new type of transplant, also called a **nonmyeloablative stem cell transplant (NST)**, "mini-transplant," and "transplant-lite," is now being performed in many centers. It is an allogeneic transplant with less toxicity. Only part of the patient's bone marrow is destroyed by chemotherapy, which results in mixed **chimerism**, or the presence of both patient and donor cells together in the bone marrow. Donor cells then kill the patient's cancer cells, and often the patient's bone marrow is transformed to be identical to the donor's. When this happens, the patient's new cells are referred to as a **full donor chimera**. Mini-allogeneic transplants use less radiation and/or chemotherapy and therefore can be successfully used in older patients (up to 75 years of age).

PART TWO

Before the Transplant: Logistics and Work-Up

How do I find a doctor who is right for me?

More . . .

Practical Tips for Managing Treatment

17. How do I find a doctor who is right for me?

Gracy's comment:

I grew up in an Asian culture in which hospitals and clinics are seen as "bad luck," so I stayed away from hospitals as much as I could. Before I fell ill, I thought doctors dressed the same, looked the same, and must all work the same. But after the transplant procedure, I realized that doctors are far from being the same. I truly believe that my experience with post-BMT recovery would have been so much more difficult (or maybe impossible) had I not had a caring doctor as my primary oncologist.

One of the most crucial decisions you will make is who will conduct your treatment. Some doctors see you as a number and use body language to show that your appointment is over and it's time for them to see the next patient. Some doctors, however, take time to listen, and hug you when you burst into tears and are feeling scared. A good doctor makes a life-and-death difference before, during, and after the BMT procedure. So how do you evaluate the doctor? Here are some tips:

A good doctor makes a life-and-death difference before, during, and after the BMT procedure.

- Does your doctor take time to explain the BMT procedure and address all your questions and concerns?
- Does he or she address all of the consequences and side effects of the procedure?
- Does he or she provide resources that can help you get mental as well as physical support while you're going through the aggressive chemotherapy and BMT procedure?
- Most importantly, does he or she exhibit the technical expertise that wins your trust and confidence?

Remember, each patient is different, so a doctor who does not take the time to get to know *you* may not be as helpful to you as one who does. A paint-by-numbers approach *could* still get the job done ... but you are likely to get better results from a doctor who pays attention to the specifics of your case, your psychological state, type of personality, survival skills, and so forth.

Post BMT is the most sensitive time during the entire BMT procedure because it represents the possibility of a new healthy life. This is all that you are waiting for. A good doctor will track your recovery through various post transplant appointments and procedures, take gradual steps to get you off numerous medications, and be available to help you whenever you encounter post-transplant side effects.

You are not alone. There are many people who have undergone transplant and want to help others. In the Appendix that follows Question 100, we provide useful web sites, phone numbers, and addresses to help you find hospitals and doctors, financial aid, and sources of information and assistance. Another good resource is the social worker of your transplant unit, who will work with you to make sure that you are returning to a safe, stable environment—a clean house and available family members or friends who can help you through this difficult process. If such an environment does not exist in your home, the social worker will help you to arrange for an alternative place to stay. The social worker will also help you to deal with health insurance, disability plans, transportation, and other important details that might be difficult for you to handle on your own. For detailed information on resources available to transplant patients, please refer to the Appendix at the end of the book.

18. Why is my bone marrow transplant doctor going to be so important?

Gracy's comment:

Your bone marrow transplant doctor plays a vital part before, during, and after the BMT procedure. An experienced transplant doctor will know how to prepare you physically as well as psychologically to reduce anxiety and pain.

There was a time following diagnosis when my husband and I were standing on the edge of hell. We knew about medical science and had learned about cancer and survival tables, but the future still looked grim. Through clear communication of compassion and caring, my bone marrow transplant doctor lifted us away from that abyss and set us down on firm ground. My doctor's personal style in working with me resulted in my fear draining away from me over time.

I was fortunate to have a bone marrow transplant doctor who is not only highly trained in her profession, but also encouraging and supportive. She inspired me to seek a place in my soul where the body and mind can mend. She is capable of touching another human with her heart as well as her hand to bring peace, as well as healing.

19. What is involved in the pre-transplant evaluation?

Pre-transplant evaluation is extensive and must be done to determine whether you are eligible for this difficult procedure. Cardiac, renal, pulmonary, and hepatic (liver) tests will be done to determine how your major organs are functioning. Test results must meet certain criteria in order for you to be eligible. Your doctor will do comprehensive serologic (blood) testing to make sure you have no active infections and to determine your past exposure to certain viral infections such as CMV. **Bone marrow aspiration biopsy** is done before the autologous stem cell transplant to determine whether your disease is in the bone marrow. A dental exam is performed to make sure you have no active cavities or infections. This should include a full set of mouth x-rays. Your dentist should make dental repairs before your transplant.

Bone marrow aspiration biopsy a procedure in which a needle is inserted into the center of a bone, usually the hip, to remove a small amount of bone marrow for microscopic examination.

20. Why is social history evaluation so important?

Transplantation is a very complicated procedure and requires social support; people must be available to help you during and after the procedure, as you probably will not be able to do many things for yourself. If you have no social support, many transplant centers will not perform the procedure, especially if you are having an allogeneic transplant. Also, the transplant center must be sure that you are willing to do what is absolutely necessary to maintain your health during and after the transplant. If you're not compliant, the expensive resources and efforts of the transplant team are wasted. The transplant cannot succeed without active effort from the patient to *make* it work by avoiding infection and limiting use of alcohol, cigarettes, and illegal drugs. A social worker will do the social evaluation that will include an educational and work history, smoking and alcohol use history, and employment and family history.

There must be people available to help you during and after the procedure.

21. What is involved in pre-transplant work-up?

Pre-transplant work-up
tests and evaluations that determine whether the patient is capable of handling a transplant.

During your **pre-transplant work-up**, a team of physicians will carefully evaluate your medical history to make sure that the procedure is appropriate for you. They will decide whether an autologous or allogeneic transplant will be performed and what conditioning will be used. They will consider all toxicities and weigh the benefits against the potential risks. After you have received full and detailed information, you will need to sign a consent form stating that you are authorizing this procedure. Signing the **informed consent** tells the doctors that you have been given enough information to make an informed decision about the transplant and understand what the transplant involves, so if there is anything about the procedure that you do not understand, you should ask questions. Do not sign the form until you are satisfied that you know what will happen.

Informed consent
a process in which all risks and complications of a procedure or treatment are explained to a patient before the procedure is done.

Before the transplant you will undergo a battery of tests to assess your overall organ function. These include functional tests on the heart, kidneys, liver, and lungs as well as a test for infections such as hepatitis. Your dentist should also perform an examination to make sure you have no infectious problems. The transplant coordinator will contact your insurance company to make sure that the transplant will be paid for in full.

A thorough work-up before the transplant procedure allows your doctor to review the state of all your vital organs (lung, heart, liver, and kidneys) before your transplant. This information will also be used as a basis for comparison after your transplant. Although it may be inconvenient, it is important to have all of these tests before your transplant.

22. Who handles the logistics of this whole process?

Gracy's comment:

If you are serious about surviving, you will become your own Director of Logistics. You need to coordinate your treatment, no matter how good the healthcare system, your BMT team, or the hospital with which they are affiliated. Your treatment involves a large number of people spread across multiple departments within a hospital or hospitals. The larger the institution, the more complex the treatment and the greater the opportunities for slip-ups. This is true for any type of large organization. Your job is to verify with everyone what the current plan is and who is going to do what, and to follow up to confirm everything. If you have the proper attitude about using the BMT to kill the cancer, you will love this job. You are the only person truly qualified for this role. Only ***you*** *know when you have had a blood test, met with a specialist outside the BMT team, or begun taking a new medication. The team thinks you have done these things because they are part of the plan, but they don't* ***know*** *that each step was actually performed.* ***You*** *know you have done them because you were present for each and every one.*

If you have a great team, they will encourage you in this role. Your transplant coordinator can only schedule appointments for you—she cannot walk over to a particular department on the day of your appointment to make sure it happens. You are not the BMT team's only patient. It is too human to let things fall between the cracks. It is up to you as the patient to take the attitude that it's ***your*** *job to catch the mistakes before they find that crack. It is an* *example of superior patient attitude to figure out better ways of doing things within your treatment.*

I am going to use outpatient medications as an example of being a creative Director of Logistics. I was taking over 10 different medications when I came home from the hospital. At the time, my health coverage limited me to a 30-day supply of each medication. I had to pay a $5.00 co-pay on each one. I tried picking up the medications at the hospital pharmacy initially. This pharmacy was always busy, and it shared a waiting room with another department within the hospital. On every visit I felt uncomfortable because the waiting room was full of sick people, some of whom had to be infectious—and the wait was long. Sitting around in a room full of sick people is not a smart thing to do if your immune system is still weak. I stopped going to the hospital pharmacy and started using the drug store near my house. I still could only get a 30-day supply at a time and had to pay the $5.00 co-pay. Subsequently, I discovered that I could order most of the medications from an online pharmacy affiliated with my HMO. When I ordered online I could get a 60- to 90-day supply each time and the co-pay was lower. But the only reason I found out about this option was that I was constantly trying to figure out better ways of doing things. It can pay off in more than just money and time. This kind of action had a strong impact on my self-esteem.

THE MONEY TRAIL

23. Why is my health insurer so important?

Once the initial evaluation shows that you are medically a potential candidate for stem cell transplant, a financial screening must take place before any further testing is done. A written statement of your specific benefits and the willingness of the payor (in most cases, your insurance company) to apply those benefits to your proposed treatment must be obtained before the transplant procedure can start. In order to obtain this statement, your transplant physician must give the payor a detailed history of your disease and justification for a transplant procedure. The payor also usually needs a "letter of necessity." They will want to determine other financial resources that you have available to cover treatment costs and additional living expenses during the stem cell transplant procedure.

Hopefully, you have some kind of group health insurance. The weaker your health insurance, the fewer options you have available to you, and the less influence you have on decisions—and ultimately the less likely you are to get through this. All of the horror stories you hear about people who are not insured can become very real if you do not plan ahead.

There are, however, places you can turn to for help if you don't have insurance. If you have been working and contributing to Social Security, there is a program that provides disability payments (see Question 26). There are also a number of government agencies, nonprofit organizations, and financial services companies that can help you manage the costs of your treatment (see Appendix). Don't forget that you can also ask the hospital social worker to help you find financial assistance.

There are, however, places you can turn to for help if you don't have insurance.

Ask the hospital social worker to help you find financial assistance.

Gracy's comment:

The cold facts are that the bigger the group coverage plan you belong to, the more likely the healthcare insurer will not block your attempts to save your life. BMT and everything that goes with it is very, very expensive. We are talking about hundreds of thousands of dollars if you add up everything, including the extended hospital stay in a private room. In these days of everyone trying to reduce health costs, patients who need very expensive treatment like the BMT are a great place for insurers to cut costs.

As hard as it is to believe, there are actually people in the United States who have health insurance and need a BMT, but get refused by their health insurance program. This usually happens to people who have individual rather than group coverage. Within the group coverage category, it can happen to you when you belong to a covered group that has a small number of members because your employer is not that big. Big companies with large numbers of employees in group coverage plans have a great deal of influence on the decisions that their health insurers make. Small companies have less influence, and individual policyholders who are not part of a group are in a bad situation.

The insurer will not tell you that the BMT is going to take too big a bite out of the bottom line for them this year. Rather, the insurer will question whether the BMT is really justifiable from a medical point of view. Perhaps they will want you to get a second opinion. All the time the old cancer clock is ticking. When you hardly have enough energy to get to the bathroom from the living room because of your current treatment, you are expected to fight your insurer's rejection of the BMT. If you have picked a good oncologist, letters from him or her and from other cancer doctors can make the insurer reverse their decision. There have been cases in which people take the insurer to court. The problem is that if your oncologist thinks that you need a BMT, you are likely to be dead before your day in court.

John and I were covered through his group health insurance with the Public Employees Retirement System (PERS) of the State of California. His health coverage was with the California Pacific Care HMO program. Our healthcare provider was the University of California, San Diego Healthcare (UCSD Healthcare). I can only say good things about the way I was treated. PERS has a great deal of influence with all healthcare insurers affiliated with it because of the massive number of current and retired State of California employees. Pacific Care did not give us any trouble whatsoever during the entire process. UCSD Healthcare took care of all my cancer care, including the BMT, pre-transplant work-up, and extended post-transplant care.

Even so, there were some snags: for instance, my oncologist wanted some tests performed on my blood following the BMT. These tests examined my blood cells at the molecular level to ensure that in the months following the BMT the leukemia was not trying to make a comeback. That is, the test would look inside my blood cells to see if a particular chromosomal translocation (I think 4/11) was present or not. The test had to be performed at a BMT research center in Minnesota because very few institutions perform such a test. Pacific Care requested that the oncologist provide them with written justification for this test. Once Pacific Care received and reviewed the justification, the expense of the tests was approved. I am still getting these tests and am so grateful that they continue to come back negative. The test on a molecular level can detect recurrence of leukemia at a very early stage and allow successful retreatment by donor leukocyte infusion.

With all the other things that were happening in my life at that time, I cannot imagine how my outcome could have differed if John and I had to fight every step of the way to get coverage from our health insurer.

24. Isn't there someone who can help me manage my transplant?

Gracy's comment:

Following the news about BMT, I received a very warm greeting from a bone marrow transplant team consisting of an attending/staff physician, a physician fellow, consulting physician, physician assistant/nurse practitioner, registered nurse, clinical care partner, clinic nurse/case manager, social worker, and dietitian. The most important team member, in my view, was my case manager (transplant coordinator), who was my link to the physician and the rest of the team (see Questions 21 and 22). My case manager was also the one who provided me with a calendar of BMT-related events and procedures to keep me on track.

Ultimately, I'm the one who was responsible for managing, tracking, and meeting each appointment necessary to fight the "last battle" of my life. I treated the doctor's schedule as my schedule. I dedicated myself full-time to meet that schedule. When my body was too tired to lift even one finger, my determination to live kicked in, and it motivated me to make just one more appointment. I realized that my will to live and spiritual strength greatly increased my chance of survival.

25. Am I going to go broke?

Gracy's comment:

In this culture just about every decision you make has to be evaluated on the money scale. It is so difficult to shift your perspective on this. I can't say I know much detail about the afterlife, but I don't think you need credit cards. John and I have both attained what we have by working hard. Our families are not wealthy. Even though we had great health insurance, our fight has been a financial disaster. An accountant would look over our financial history for the last 3 years and burst into tears. At times it is depressing to think about what was and what is today in financial terms. As soon as my mind starts moving in this direction, reality kicks in. What good is a BMW, a remodeled bathroom, or a two-week vacation if you are in a place where there are no streets?

From the day I was diagnosed with leukemia, John started planning for any route that our trip might go.

During the conditioning for the BMT, John retired from his job to become my caretaker. He drove me to the chemotherapy sessions, visited me as much as possible when I was in the hospital, and took care of me when I came home after the BMT. Not everyone would do this. Not everyone could do this. It is a type of "letting go" that is extremely hard for people dedicated to career and the fruits of career.

When John's mother was diagnosed with breast cancer some years ago, he continued working on his Ph.D. and full-time job. When he could, he would drive to his mother's home and check on how she was doing. He was told that everything was going fine and that she was in remission. One day he received a call from his sister. His mother had died. The cancer had spread throughout her body and despite the best efforts of the medical people there was little to do but treat the pain. His mother had not wanted him to know how bad things were. This personal experience with his mother's cancer caused John to think a long time about how he might have done things differently.

If the treatment outcomes were poor and my prognosis nose-dived, the plan was to hit the road. John was going to take me to Taiwan to be with my family, and we would spend the rest of our days together at my family's home. Once I was gone, he would start to think about what he would do next. Since he is a hopelessly romantic person, you can figure out what his plans were at the time.

Today we are starting all over again. We have each other and a whole new group of dreams for the future. We owe so much money that it would take a California state lottery win to get us on the plus side again. As bad as the money situation sounds, it does not bother us. This is a Godzilla-sized change in attitude for both of us. We have less money and more debt, but are so much happier than we were before. It's better to be broke than dead!

26. Can Social Security Disability Insurance help?

Gracy's comment:

Since I had been in the workplace for a number of years, Social Security Disability Insurance (SSDI) covered me. I contacted the local Social Security Administration office and sent John down to pick up the paperwork. Once the forms had been filled out and signed by my oncologist, we submitted them to Social Security. I started receiving my checks for Social Security disability shortly after that. You hear from time to time how the federal government does not do this or that correctly. If you find yourself in the same situation I was in, you will discover that the Social Security Administration is something that the government did right. I have nothing but praise for the people working in that organization. The SSDI program helped me when I was not fit at all to work. When I was well enough to return to work, Social Security Administration put me in a "trial-work" program that is designed to provide incentives and a smooth transition to bring a formerly disabled person, like myself, back to the workplace. Please contact your local Social Security Administration office to find out more about these programs (see the Appendix).

27. What about private disability insurance?

Gracy's comment:

My employer carried disability insurance for everyone who worked at the company. This disability insurance came in handy after I took leave from work to deal with the cancer. If you have disability insurance, you might want to look very closely at the small print in the policy. In our case, the disability insurance payout was calculated as a percentage of what I had been making monthly on the job. Our disability insurer deducted any state disability payments or social security disability payments from that monthly amount. The result was that what seemed like a significant amount of money when you read the policy became much less significant when the rules hidden in the fine print were applied. It really was our own fault for not looking more closely at the policy. When everything is going well, you do not even think to check these things out.

Our experience with the disability insurance company (one of the biggest in the world) was not as positive as it could have been. Insurance companies tend to see the disabled insured as a major income drain and a potential fraud case. There was a huge gap between when my check from work stopped and the insurance disability check started to arrive. I think they might have been afraid of overpaying me. Hence, they waited until I applied for the state of California and Social Security Administration disability so that they could figure out how much to deduct before sending me the first disability check. During the illness itself, they would call or write constantly to make sure that I was not recovered enough to return to work. Here I was, diagnosed with a very deadly form of leukemia, and the disability insurance people were constantly badgering us with forms for the oncologist to fill out to prove that I was not able to go back to work yet.

I am thankful that in the middle of all this, John and I managed to develop and sustain a sense of humor. The idea of a person whose immune system has been totally destroyed being asked to verify that she cannot go back to work was so funny that we began to think that someone at the disability insurance company had a sense of humor too!

28. Am I eligible for state disability insurance?

Gracy's comment:

Individual states vary in the amount of disability insurance they provide. Since I had been working for some time, the state of California was able to provide me with monthly disability payments. The payments are calculated based on the number of months you have worked. I did not have to apply directly for the state disability insurance. The human resources department of the company I worked for did that for me.

29. What is a durable power of attorney for health care?

Durable power of attorney for health care

a legal document naming a specific person as the patient's healthcare decision maker should the patient become too ill to make his or her own decisions.

A **durable power of attorney for health care** is a document that allows you to name a person (relative or friend) who can make all medical decisions for you if you cannot speak for yourself, including authorizing or refusing any medical treatment. (This person is sometimes referred to as a "health care proxy.") Your attending physician will activate the durable power of attorney for health care because he or she, as the physician who is in charge of your care, is considered to be the person best able to tell whether you are no longer capable of making or communicating decisions. In the state of California, if you don't have someone to appoint as your agent, then a Natural Death Act Declaration will take effect if you become terminally ill or permanently unconscious and are no longer able to make decisions about life-sustaining treatment. However, different states have different laws for these circumstances. For more information, please discuss your concerns with your physician and social workers, or consult an attorney; any of these individuals should be able to provide information about your state's rules regarding healthcare proxies and power-of-attorney documents.

FINDING A DONOR

30. What is involved in the process of finding a donor?

The potential donor for allogeneic transplant can be a sibling, an unrelated matched donor, or, less frequently, parents or children. An additional source of stem cells can be unrelated cord blood where the stem cells are taken from the repository.

The search for an unrelated donor may take 3 to 6 months; such donors are generally found through computer searches of national registries such as the National Bone Marrow Donor Program (see Question 31; contact information is in the Appendix), which has records of hundreds of individuals' HLA information. If a potential donor is found, blood samples are taken from both the patient and potential donor, and special tests are carried out to confirm the HLA match. The process takes about 2 to 3 weeks to complete. Then the donor is examined and cleared medically by the physician.

The search for an unrelated donor may take 3 to 6 months.

31. What is the National Bone Marrow Donor Program (NMDP)?

The NMDP is a federally funded program that was created in 1968 to help find matching bone marrow donors for patients worldwide. Fewer than 25% of patients have a matching sibling donor, and therefore many patients require unrelated donor transplants. The NMDP coordinates searches throughout the United

States as well other countries. NMDP tries to maintain bone marrow samples that are representative of diverse ethnic populations. However, some ethnic groups, such as African-Americans and Asians, are underrepresented. This means that the likelihood of a person in these ethnic groups finding an unrelated donor is much lower than for other ethnic groups that are widely represented in the registry, as some of the HLA factors that determine a good match differ from one race to another. NMDP makes a constant effort to recruit donors from these minority groups.

NMDP is a large registry with several million potential donors. These are volunteer donors who agreed to have their blood analyzed and typed for potential use in BMT. NMDP can also connect with the registries of other countries by computer.

32. How does someone become a donor? Are donors volunteers? Can anyone be a donor?

All registries require that donors be volunteers, who may not be coerced into agreeing to donate marrow in any way. The National Marrow Donor Program requires that the potential donor be an adult between the ages of 18 and 55, be in good general health, not be excessively overweight, have read a pamphlet called "What you should know about being a donor," and have a general understanding about what it means to become a donor. The donor must also understand the potential for transmitting infections, such as HIV and hepatitis, through blood, marrow, and plasma donation. The factors that would exclude someone from being a donor include substance abuse, cancer, sickle cell anemia, B-thalassemia major, active asthma, diabetes, heart problems, HIV, or hepatitis B and C. You, as a patient, will never be able to become a donor.

33. How is a donor screened?

Potential allogeneic stem cell donors undergo HLA typing. Once an allogeneic donor is found, he or she must give a complete medical history and undergo a review of systems (a history of symptoms related to any organ or system, such as respiratory, cardiovascular, digestive, etc.) and a physical examination. Specifically, the donor will be screened for history of chronic or serious illness, history of bleeding tendencies, cancer history, transfusion history, adverse anesthesia reaction, current medications, allergies, history of HIV or hepatitis, and, in females, history of previous pregnancies. Donors with a history of HIV or cancer will be rejected. If several donors are available for a specific transplant, donors of the same sex as the patient and CMV–negative donors are preferred.

34. Why is HLA match important?

The better the match between your bone marrow and the bone marrow that is being transplanted into you, the fewer complications you will have. Since the entire process is difficult, even in the best of circumstances, you want to do all you can to make sure that you have the fewest complications. A good match also lessens the chance that you will experience GVHD.

GVHD symptoms can come in as many forms as there are people. Gracy had itching on various parts of her body. Strange rashes showed up on her skin. The important thing is to be in tune with your own body and to be aware of what is not normal for you. If you communicate well with your doctor, he or she can prescribe drugs to lessen the GVHD symptoms.

Gracy's comment:

In my case, even though the match was excellent, there were still some graft-versus-host disease (GVHD) side effects. Get used to saying "GVHD" because you are going to hear it a great deal. The new bone marrow that you receive from someone else is the graft. You are the host. When the graft and the host are adjusting to one another you experience symptoms. People will refer to these manifestations of the "adjusting" as GVHD.

35. Who is the best donor?

An HLA-matched sibling—one who shares most or all of the same antigens as the patient—is usually the best donor. In general, sibling donors tend to be close in age to the patient, and a young donor is better than an older donor. Donors between 20 and 50 years of age probably provide the same quality of stem cells, although this has not been studied in detail in humans. Donors older than 60 years of age may have a difficult time donating enough stem cells. Male donors are better than female donors who have been pregnant. Different tests are done to find out whether the donor is HLA-matched with the patient, and the ideal donor matches the patient in all of the criteria. In some instances, six criteria are used, and a perfect match is called a 6/6 match; in others, ten criteria are used, and a 10/10 match is desirable. Transplants can be done with 5/6 or 9/10 matches, but they are riskier than perfect matches. Oddly enough, children and parents of the patient are rarely good donors. There is usually a significant HLA mismatching (3/6). Only occasionally are children a 5/6 match, and they can be used for transplant when no other donors are available.

36. How is the donor's stem cell collection performed?

Bone Marrow Harvest

If you are having an autologous transplant, you will be your own donor and will have your own stem cells and bone marrow collected. If you will receive stem cells from a donor, he or she will undergo a bone marrow or stem cell collection. Bone marrow harvest is a surgical procedure in which a needle is inserted into the hipbone many times in order to obtain 1–1.5 liters of bone marrow (diluted with blood). Marrow rich in stem cells will be withdrawn and stored until the transplant. During the surgery, the donor will be anesthetized and will not feel any pain, although the area of the surgery may be sore for several days after the procedure. A detailed description of this procedure is given in Question 4.

Peripheral Blood Stem Cell Collection

Peripheral stem cells can be collected from the bloodstream. The process of collecting stem cells in the blood is called **peripheral blood stem cell (PBSC)** collection. Like stem cells from the blood, PBSCs are able to move to the bone marrow and make red blood cells, white blood cells, and platelets. The bloodstream only has a small number of stem cells, so a protein called granulocyte-colony stimulating factor (G-CSF) will be used to help move more stem cells out from the donor's bone marrow into his or her peripheral blood. Once they are in the blood, they will be collected by a process called **apheresis**. Through a central line placed in the donor's vein (see Question 51) before the procedure, he or she will be connected to the apheresis

Peripheral blood stem cell (PBSC)
stem cells that circulate in the blood.

Apheresis
collection of stem cells from the blood.

machine and blood will be circulated through a cell separator. The stem cells will then be removed and stored until the transplant. The rest of the blood will be returned to the donor. Apheresis is painless, and each collection lasts 3 to 6 hours. An average of 2 to 5 collections are needed to get enough stem cells. The collection process is essentially the same for allogeneic and autologous transplant.

Gracy's comment:

My sister Brenda and I would arrive at the apheresis room around 8:30 each morning. I watched the technician attach two tubes to Brenda, one on each arm (her veins were big enough and she did not need a central catheter placed). When the machine was turned on, the live stem cells from Brenda's body were captured in a bag. I watched Brenda's blood being pumped from a tube in her left arm, through the apheresis machine, and back to her body through the right arm. A bag attached to the apheresis machine held the stems cells that the machine filtered out during this process. Being a healthy young woman and stimulated by a few shots of G-CSF (one shot daily during procedure), Brenda's body produced extra stem cells. I later came to refer to these extra stems cells as my "stream of life." The same routine was repeated for several days in a row. Each session lasted 4 to 5 hours. During each apheresis, Brenda had to stay very still and could not move or go to the bathroom. So, I thank God that the clinic provided a comfortable environment. This was done by having a comfortable bed for her to lie on during the procedure and a television (VCR ready) to decrease the boredom. The only impact that Brenda felt from the procedure was the soreness in her arms where the IV needles had been attached.

37. What is involved in stem cell collection and infusion?

The hematopoietic stem cells are collected at the site where the donor is registered. The donor is given growth factors, such as granulocyte-colony stimulating factor (G-CSF) or granulocyte macrophage-colony stimulating factor (GM-CSF), or chemotherapy (cyclophosphamide) to "mobilize" stem cells—that is, to induce them to leave the bone marrow and enter the blood. The collection of these stem cells with an apheresis machine takes about 1 to 3 days. The donor rests on a reclining chair while apheresis is taking place. Blood is filtered through a cell separator via the catheter, frozen, and stored, and the stored cells are flown to your transplant center. The stem cells are then infused into your blood through the venous catheter like a blood product. This process takes place over several hours and has no side effects. Minor allergic reactions can occur but they are rare and usually reversible, and the physician and nursing staff will watch you carefully for signs of problems.

38. Can I meet my unrelated donor?

The National Marrow Donor Program (NMDP) protects the identity of the donor for one year post transplant. After that, they can reveal the identity of the donor if the donor has given them permission to do so. Sometimes the donor and the patient arrange a meeting, share experiences, and a few donors and patients develop long-term friendships. It is a matter of whether you wish to meet the donor and whether the donor is open to this meeting. Some donors, however, prefer to remain anonymous, and this wish must be respected.

It is a matter of whether you wish to meet the donor and whether the donor is open to this meeting.

39. What is CD34 count?

Surface marker

a protein on the surface of a cell that helps identify the cell.

Flow cytometry

a test done on cancerous tissues that shows the aggressiveness of the tumor.

CD34 is a **surface marker** (a protein on the surface of a cell) for the human hematopoietic stem cell. In 1980, a technique called **flow cytometry** became useful in determining how many cells contained this marker, information that is essential for transplantation. About 3 to 5 million cells with the CD34 marker are required per kilogram of body weight for successful transplantation. A CD34+ cell count below 1 million cells/kg may mean prolonged neutropenia and a greater chance of infections, or even failure of the transplant.

PART THREE

Caring for Your Body and Mind

What is a “special ventilation system”?
Is this something I’ll need in my home?

How do I find the time to manage my treatment?

More . . .

40. *What is a "special ventilation system"? Is this something I'll need in my home?*

Air quality is of utmost importance for patients receiving full allogeneic transplant, who tend to be severely immunocompromised. This is especially important in old buildings and warm or humid climates, conditions that encourage fungal growth. The quality of filtration systems ranges from no filtration, standard filtration, and high-efficiency particulate air (HEPA) filtration to the most effective form, laminar air flow (LAF) filtration. Most air-conditioning units are equipped with standard filtration, which can filter particles of about 10–15 microns (one-thousandth of a millimeter). It is better than no filtration at all, but is probably not good enough for an immunocompromised person. The next method, HEPA filtration, is better: it will remove particles of 0.3 microns 99.9% of the time, providing considerably superior air quality. LAF filtration takes this one step further: it uses HEPA-filtered air to create a particle-free, sterile environment by moving air through a filtration system and sending the particles on an airstream away from the patient. The LAF room is usually fully enclosed and kept under constant positive pressure in order to prevent contaminated outside air from coming into the room. People entering these rooms must be completely sterile—that is, wearing gowns, masks, a cap, and sterile gloves—so that the room remains uncontaminated.

The cost of the specialized equipment used in LAF systems is enormous, so naturally they are used in hospitals or cancer centers, not private homes. If your hospital has such a room and your doctors feel you need to be in it, then you will have to stay there as long as your doctors think it necessary. The use of LAF rooms varies from center to center. HEPA-filtered rooms provide clean air without the restrictions of the LAF rooms (gowns, masks, caps, and sterile gloves). In a HEPA-filtered room, the air is exchanged about 10 to 15 times an hour. Positive air pressure causes air to flow from the room into the hallway so that contaminated air can't come into the room. The air in the hallway in a HEPA-filtered unit will be exchanged about six times an hour, with air flowing from the unit into the adjacent area of the hospital.

Standard HEPA filtration systems are available to private homeowners and are generally supplied to people with respiratory problems or allergies to dust. If your doctor does not tell you to use the high-quality filtration of a hospital, you probably don't need one of these systems. If you can afford to get one, however, having one will give you the benefits of clean air that has fewer particles in it.

41. How do I find the time to manage my treatment?

Gracy's comment:

As you read through this, you might be thinking to yourself that you just don't have the time to handle all these tasks—coordinating your care, hunting for the best deals on medications, becoming an expert on your disease and its treatment. All of this can take years. One aspect of developing the right attitude is coming to terms with your conception of time. Time in the sense you knew it before diagnosis is gone. You have been transported to the "BMT galaxy" where time is compressed. When you were diagnosed with the cancer, or aplastic anemia, or whatever it is that has brought you to the transplant table, the universe was giving you a hint. The hint is that your time is more than likely going to be different than other people's. You are going to be one of those people who thinks of life in terms of quality rather than quantity. Most people walk around acting like they will live forever and thinking little about making the most of the time they have. You are lucky enough to know that it is not forever and you are going to have to respond appropriately.

The more you focus every fiber of your being on having a successful BMT, the better your chances of expanding your time. By dedicating every ounce of your physical and spiritual energy to the BMT, you will experience in months what some people take years to know: the joy of living each day as if it were your last, of making each moment count. How else in a life can you go from being so weak you can't lift your arm to feeling that you could lift the whole world up on your shoulders?

42. What is a survival table?

If you decide to go to the Internet to try to obtain information on your cancer and the bone marrow transplant, eventually you will find survival tables. Survival tables keep track of how long people who develop a particular disease survive after they are diagnosed. For example, a survival table might display a graph that tracks 40 people who developed acute lymphoblastic leukemia (ALL) and show how many were still alive after 3, 5, or 10 years. Some of the tables control for age, race, sex, treatment type, and other factors. In theory, if you were an African-American man over the age of 50 undergoing a given type of BMT, you could look at such a table to get an idea of how long men of your age and race generally survive.

If you want to get even more technical, you can go online and visit cancer research web sites where they track groups of people who not only have a particular cancer but also exhibit certain **genetic** abnormalities specific to that cancer. This can have a significant impact on **prognosis**; having acute lymphoblastic leukemia is bad enough, but having acute lymphoblastic leukemia accompanied by what is called 4/11 gene translocation makes the prognosis even worse.

Genetic

refers to the inherited pattern located in genes for certain characteristics.

Prognosis

a prediction of the course of the disease—the future prospects for the patient's life and welfare.

A comparison of survival rates for patients undergoing a bone marrow transplant compared to patients who received high-dose chemotherapy followed by low-dose chemotherapy on an ongoing basis is a common research paper topic. Treatment of patients, to a researcher, goes beyond simply keeping these patients alive—it also gives the researcher information that helps him or her determine how effective your treatment is for people with a certain disease. Thus, the results of your treatment are combined with treatment results of others receiving the same treatment. These group results are compared to another group of people who received a different treatment. The hope is that by comparing treatment outcomes, doctors and scientists will discover the most effective way to combat the illness.

Gracy's comment:

I think the survival tables are useful for researchers, insurance companies, and others, but useless for people like us. Every human is unique, so expecting to look at a survival table and gain any predictive value on the nature of your future is illogical. The tables classify people on general characteristics such as sex, age, race, treatment type, and so forth. There may be people out there who are similar to you in terms of sex, age, race, and treatment type, but if you have been around for any amount of time on earth, you know that you are different in more important, subtle ways. The tables do not classify by attitude, how loved you are, the quality of your soul, or your relationship with God, to mention a few items. If you want to get depressed, then go ahead and look at the tables. If you want to get well, do something that strengthens your attitude, increases how loved you are, expands your reserve of soul, or allows you feel the presence of God.

If you want to get depressed, then go ahead and look at the tables.

43. What can I do to improve my chances of survival?

How you come out of the bone marrow transplant depends on the skill of the bone marrow transplant medical team, your attitude, and a good match for bone marrow. If the bone marrow team is working out of a hospital that is one of the national centers for bone marrow transplant, and the doctor leading the team is very aggressive in cancer treatment and wants to kill your cancer, you have the first base covered. If you have developed a firm attitude that allows you to focus all your energy on actively participating in the bone marrow transplant with an unwavering belief in success, you have reachedsecond base. Third base, finding a bone marrow donor who is a good match for your body, can be a difficult one to cover.

70% of the people who need a bone marrow transplant cannot find a donor whose bone marrow is a good match.

Over 70% of the people who need a bone marrow transplant cannot find a donor whose bone marrow is a good match for their own. Imagine being in that situation. The doctors know that they can save your life, but they can't find the bone marrow to save it with. Why is it so hard to find a donor? The closer the donor is to a clone of you, an exact copy, the better the chances that the new bone marrow and your body will be able to live with one another. The further away you get from an exact copy of you, the greater the chances that your body and the new bone marrow will try to kill one another (transplant rejection).

In some cases, as described in Questions 11–13, doctors take out some of your own bone marrow, purge it of cancer, kill all the bone marrow remaining in you, and reintroduce your purged bone marrow. You might think this is the best way to go. Unfortunately, if your cancer is very severe or of a certain type, this is not an option.

When medical people talk of a bone marrow match between you and another person, they can be very specific. Your bone marrow is compared to another person's bone marrow using a number of criteria, as discussed in Questions 14 and 34. The more criteria that match each other, the better the chances of success in getting the donor bone marrow to work inside your body. The best match for bone marrow would be an identical twin. The next best match would be a fraternal twin. From there we move to a brother or sister. If none of these works, perhaps it will be possible to find a person unrelated to you who matches.

The point is that the less the donor bone marrow matches your own bone marrow, the greater the chances of complications due to rejection. Complications take the form of mild illness, serious illness, and sometimes death. The hard fact is that if you are at the point where you need a transplant, then you're likely facing certain death already if you do *not* undertake the transplant. It is worth taking the risk when you consider the alternative.

44. My illness has been hard on my loved ones. What can I do to help those around me right now?

Gracy's comment:

When I was made aware that BMT transplant was the only chance I had to defeat my cancer, I felt hurt, confused, depressed, and helpless. It wasn't long before I realized that these emotions were like highly contagious germs. They not only infected me but also infected my husband and all of those who truly loved and cared about me. I think it is fair to say that I should be the last one to complain about the emotional distress because I was preoccupied through the entire treatment. But those who try to use work or a job to create the same effect (occupy the mind) could be less successful and end up being more hurt, confused, and depressed than I was.

I did several things that were helpful to those around me. I communicated clearly when I talked about the status of my treatment. I named specific chores when I needed help. I made arrangements assuming the worst while maintaining my most upbeat attitude. I recognized and gave others room to feel their pain.

45. Who can I talk to about this experience—someone who will really understand?

The best people to talk to about the transplant experience are the members of your BMT team. If you have done your homework in selecting the best oncologist, team, and hospital, you will be surrounded by opportunities to get your questions answered. These people live the BMT routine and love to share what they know with others. At times, they will forget that you are a nonmedical person and start to speak in what seems to be a foreign language. All you have to do is be patient and continue to ask them to define their terms for you. They will not grow impatient with you unless you grow impatient with them.

Most people who have good hearts (and some of the biggest hearts are in medical people) are going to look for nonverbal clues when answering your questions. If they see that you are not taking what you hear very well, they may be less direct in the future. How much they reveal to you depends on how much you show them you can handle. If you consistently show people that you can handle direct answers without getting flustered, they will continue to give you direct answers.

If you consistently show people that you can handle direct answers without getting flustered, they will continue to give you direct answers.

You need to start and continue this dialogue with your team if you want to be an active participant in your BMT process. As an active participant, you are going to have to educate yourself in the language that the team uses to communicate. That means that you listen very closely and ask questions whenever you can. This willingness to push yourself to learn by asking is one of the essential factors that make up having the right attitude. Since you and your illness are unique, as unique as every human is, only your BMT team can give you an accurate picture. It is very important for you to know where you are now and what is to come.

Once you have established good communication between you and your BMT team, you should consider speaking with other BMT patients. Ask your doctor or a nurse how to find support groups, where they meet, how to access chat rooms on the Internet, and so on.

Some of this information is provided in the Appendix. Many people have survived this ordeal, and you may benefit from meeting and talking to them. You can take the information that you have learned from your BMT team and ask questions of other, more experienced patients. They are not going to be able to answer questions about your HLA antigens, but they will be able to answer general questions. Patients are nonmedical people like you. Medical people take it for granted that sores are going to develop in your mouth when your immune system has been wiped out. You might think a sore in the mouth means the same thing whether a medical person or a nonmedical person uses the term. Believe me, there are sores, and there are super sores. A patient who has already gone through the process can give you some information that will set your mind at ease when you develop the sores yourself.

Support Groups

When you are diagnosed, many people may start to leave your life, avoiding you for one reason or another. Some may be afraid of not knowing how to act around you. Some may be afraid that they might "get" what you have. Others may just be afraid—particularly when your disease is cancer, which frightens many people just by being mentioned. Unless you have previously had cancer yourself or someone very close to you has had it, you are as ignorant as those people who start to leave your life. The best people to ask about cancer are the people who have it themselves. They will answer your questions much better than other people because they are in the same boat as you.

Gracy's comment:

I was invited to the cancer support group meeting affiliated with the University of California, San Diego Center for Transplantation. Both my husband, John, and myself were not real excited about attending any kind of support group, much less a cancer support group. I don't apologize for it; that's just the way we were. Cancer is a great motivator. The knowledge that you are going to undergo the bone marrow transplant puts even greater spin on that motivation. We went to the meeting.

The people in the room were a snapshot of cancer. They varied from each other in the same way all Americans do. In age, sex, race, and so on, they were just like a group of folks who had been picked up off the street and dropped into that room by a big hand. They were a snapshot, too, in the sense that some were just starting the fight, some were in the middle of the fight, and a few were survivors counting their months and years of life since treatment. By watching and listening, we got an idea of what our future was going to be like.

The meeting was a mountain of information because we listened and learned a great deal of practical advice as the people talked with one another about the status of their treatment. The most important thing we learned was how different people exhibited their unique attitudes to their cancer. Some people were angry and ready to do anything to beat the hell out of the cancer. I got the impression from one woman that if she had a shotgun she would be only too pleased to blow the head off of her cancer. Some people were upset but had confidence in medical science. A few were depressed and gave the impression of being doomed. I now realize that the most important thing that John and I learned from the meeting was that there are different ways you can choose to react to cancer and its treatment. Your personal attitude about the fight is just as important as the weapons you use.

If you have cancer, get up off of your butt and go to a cancer support group meeting. Take your main sources of social support with you. They have questions and they are hurting also. You will see with your own eyes what the future holds for you. It may not be pretty, but you will be able to prepare for it. You'll get straight, practical answers to questions that have been driving you crazy. Most importantly, you will get a feel for where you fit into the scale of willingness to fight the disease.

If you don't have cancer, there are probably organizations or groups to support people who have your disease. Your doctor or case manager should be able to point you toward some helpful organizations. If not, check the Appendix at the back of the book, or you can get on the Internet and simply search on the name of your disease, perhaps limiting the search to "support groups." You'll be amazed at what's out there.

Sooner or later, however, unless you want to become a hospital groupie, you are going to have to talk with someone outside the medical team/support group universe. It is so easy to hide within your disease and the medical system. It can become very warm and cozy. However, you have to remember that your goal is to get to a place where the medical team can take care of other people and the support group can assist new folks. You have to keep one foot in the world that you want to return to eventually.

Family and Friends

How much you tell your loved ones is completely up to you. You will find out very quickly who can take it and who would rather pass. Hopefully you have a friend or lover who loves you so much that he or she is willing to listen without running—that is, running in either the physical sense of getting up and walking out the door, as very few people actually do, or running in the emotional sense, in which the mind just stops receiving information. Having such a person to talk to is great because you are going to need someone with whom you can share your feelings whose heart is in sync with your own—not so much to have someone to share information with as to have someone to share feelings with. There is going to be a lot of crying, and there is nothing wrong with crying together. In time, humor will enter the picture, and you will actually be able to laugh in situations in which others would find it inappropriate.

You are going to need someone with whom to share your feelings.

46. Will I be different after my transplant?

Gracy's comment:

It has been almost three years since my bone marrow transplant, and I'm still noticing ways in which I am different than before the transplant. These differences fall into the categories of physical, cognitive, and spiritual change. Others around me seem to have changed also. They could be responding to the change they see in me, to the new person.

I've gained weight, but I don't worry about it because increasing the pounds goes along with the successful transplant. Food tastes so much better than it did before because I developed a new appreciation for food as a result of my treatment. I have scars on my chest from where the catheters went in, but they are not large and over time I notice them less and less. My hair, fingernails, and toenails seem to grow much faster than they used to. This could be because I am eating larger quantities of healthy foods like fruits, vegetables, and grains. I take estrogen because the irradiation fried my ovaries. I was not planning on having any children before, but now it's not even a possibility. Although the chemotherapy, the irradiation, the bone marrow transplant, and the numerous drugs I've taken during the process could have impacted other organs of my body, everything has recovered—and in some cases improved.

The hardest thing to get a feel for is whether there has been a change in my cognition. Do I process information differently than I did before the bone marrow transplant? If this has changed, it would be hard for me to know because I would no longer be aware of the way I used to think about things. My husband, John, says there were phases I went through where my mental alertness and ability to process information about the world seemed different to someone like him looking at me from the outside. During the irradiation treatments, he noticed that I took a long time to respond to simple questions and that sometimes I would lose track of a conversation we were having. This was of great concern to him at the time because he was afraid it would get worse and be permanent. Even now, he claims that I am the same Gracy, but with a different flavor. A better flavor than before. Like getting married again.

After putting my body through so much pain and suffering, the spiritual side of me began to respond in a very magical way. A transformation started to take place before, during, and after the transplant. Even today, I'm still feeling the effect of this transformation. Unfortunately, this spiritual transformation is not guaranteed or a given. It is also not measurable, like some kind of weight loss program or cosmetic surgery where you can get exact snapshots of the "before" and "after." But a few things I can identify for sure: I don't take tomorrow's sunrise for granted; I make time to smell flowers in my garden; I can prioritize my day with ease; I am strong enough to say no when before I could not; I don't sweat the small stuff; I am in tune with my body and soul; and I live my days to their fullest extent.

I don't take tomorrow's sunrise for granted; I make time to smell flowers in my garden.

Listen very carefully to your body and soul throughout your transplant. You just might see the magical, spiritual transformation that I now refer to as "enlightenment."

47. Will my blood type change after the transplant?

Your blood type will not change after an autologous stem cell transplant, because your own stem cells are transplanted. However, in the case of allogeneic transplants in which the donor's blood type is different from yours, your blood type will change to that of the donor, usually after 3 months. In some cases, donor **lymphocytes** (infection-fighting white blood cells) may make antibodies to your red blood cells, and a condition called **hemolytic anemia** occurs—that is, your red blood cell count may drop because the transplanted lymphocytes attack them. This problem can be treated with prednisone until your blood type changes to that of your donor, at which point the problem will disappear. The histocompatibility (HLA) antigens will also change, and you will acquire the donor's HLA type.

Lymphocyte
white blood cell that fights infections, often found in the lymphatic system and spleen.

Hemolytic anemia
a condition arising when a patient's red blood cells are destroyed by the donor's lymphocytes.

48. How will others interpret my need for the BMT?

Most people hate like hell to be reminded that our lives are short and that we usually don't have control over when we die. Also, Western culture prepares us for assuming many roles as we move through life, but the role of being seriously ill or facing death is one for which we are never trained. Thus, folks who have a serious illness that could result in death make most people feel uncomfortable. People are uncomfortable because there are no clear rules for how to act around people like you. It does not mean that your loved ones don't like or love you anymore, only that they don't know what to do or say when they are around you. You

If some people are uncomfortable around you, look at it as a form of ignorance that is no fault of yours or theirs.

can look at it as a form of ignorance that is no fault of yours or theirs.

Having people treat you a certain way because of your health status rather than who you are as a person can be extremely hard on your sense of self. If you have not experienced discrimination in your life, this could open your eyes to feelings you might not have known could exist. These feelings can be very negative and extremely strong when you are already waist deep in profound emotions related to your treatment. If you don't cope with these feelings in a positive way up front, they could have a huge impact on your chances of getting through the treatment.

When you hear about certain groups of people being discriminated against, you might feel in your heart that it is wrong. You may feel that perhaps folks are just being overly sensitive when they talk of "discrimination," and that perhaps a change in their attitude would make them feel differently. You are going to learn what it is like to have a sixth sense. No matter what the situation, regardless of how subtle the delivery, you are going to learn to perceive when someone is responding to your health status rather than you.

Gracy's comment:

Those close to you, because they are close to you, may experience the same behavior from people. My husband described how differently people who he had known for a long time started treating him once they found out about my cancer. Some people tried their best to avoid interacting with him. Others would do their best to make their interactions with him as short as possible. A few would turn the conversation to salvation and the power of prayer, depending on their religious orientation. People who had family or friends with cancer would describe the type of cancer, the impact it had on the person, and what the outcome of the cancer experience had been. A small number of people treated the cancer like just another part of life in a direct manner. He began to feel most comfortable around people who did not know I had cancer or those who made no big thing of it. After a while he began to contemplate not telling anyone else that I had cancer.

49. Will I lose my hair?

If you have an autologous or allogeneic transplant, you will probably lose your hair within two weeks post transplant. Your hair will probably start to grow back within several weeks post transplant, depending on your chemotherapy. It will likely take several months for your hair to grow back fully. The color and texture of your hair may change—and many patients think it is better than its pre-transplant appearance. Wigs are a good option if you're uncomfortable with your appearance, and some women use scarves and caps. Some patients shave their head and acquire a new, interesting, fashionable look, although for some that may be a negative reminder of cancer therapy.

Your hair will probably start to grow back within several weeks post transplant.

Gracy's comment:

My doctors had me on chemotherapy before the transplant, both to keep me alive and to try to get my body to stabilize before we could really attack the cancer. The chemotherapy caused my hair to start falling out at a slow pace. Once they thought I was ready, we started full-body irradiation to kill every bit of cancer anywhere in my body. It also killed a lot of things that were not cancer. This is when it seemed that hair loss went from a little at a time to gone in days.

Some aspects of the cure can be as bad as the disease, but not as bad as being dead. Seeing my hair coming out in clumps in the shower, on my pillow, and on my hairbrush was enough to drive me insane. My hair was so much a part of what I saw as "me" when I looked in the mirror.

We visited a wig store and picked up a wig that made me look like a Chinese version of Tina Turner. The stores that sell wigs, and the different styles of wigs they stock, could be worth a book in themselves. John said we were going to need to have a sense of humor about this or else we were going to be crying all the time. He wanted me to get a red wig with white swirls in it. Right! Only in his dreams would I wear that wig. I selected the "Tina" wig with blond hair and black streaks in it. We also picked up some of those head caps that are supposed to hide the fact that you don't have any hair. They were comfortable, but they did not hide anything from anyone. At a certain point I got comfortable with the whole thing and stopped wearing the wig.

Eventually I lost all my hair. My hair started to slowly grow back when I got home from the hospital stay for the bone marrow transplant. Each night before we went to sleep, John would get out the magnifying glass and count the little black stubs on my skull where new hair was just starting to break the surface. Using the magnifying glass to find the stubs gives you an idea of how small they were. Over time (years) my hair grew back to the shoulder length I prefer. We believe it grew more quickly because John adopted my hair as his "crop" and kissed it and rubbed it every night to make it grow back strong and healthy.

Once you see your hair go, you can't be sure of whether it will come back again. But if it does, it can come back in variety of different forms—lighter, darker, thicker, thinner, straighter, or curlier. My sister, who was my donor, has always had thicker and curlier hair than mine. After the transplant, my hair is now thicker and curlier. Not only am I happy with the new hair, but I also feel that I have paid for it in full.

50. How will the transplant affect my energy level?

Your energy level is going to vary.

Your energy level is going to vary depending on what stage of the BMT you are in and what type of medications you are taking. The high dose chemotherapy and the full body irradiation used to prepare you for the BMT will put you on an energy roller coaster. The same is true for the first few months you are home from the hospital. By listening closely to what the BMT team advises, you can prevent yourself from hitting the lowest energy levels. This still leaves a great deal of room for ups and downs. Listening to your body and making your attitude work for you can help.

Gracy's comment:

Listening to your body is a form of awareness. Not awareness of the environment around you, but awareness of the cues your body gives when you are wearing yourself down. I think we all vary in the nature of individual cues. My cue was a general feeling of discomfort and a feeling that my eyelids were getting heavy. After experiencing extremes in energy changes for a time, I began to recognize the cues and would modify my behavior. Most of the extreme dives in energy occurred because I had not learned to look for these cues and was burning energy when I had little to spare. Another benefit of learning these cues was that I was able to identify behaviors that were draining me. Getting up too quickly and trying to walk around too fast were two behaviors that would rob me of energy very quickly.

Regardless of how aware you are of your body's warning signs, there will be times when you get totally drained no matter what you do. This goes with the territory. It is to be expected. During BMT conditioning, the very components of your body that make you strong are being killed at the same time as the cancerous cells. *Attitude* is going to allow you to give yourself as much sleep as possible. We all have ideas of what enough sleep is and how long we should be up during the day. This does not apply to you. The sooner you learn this, the better off you will be. Attitude also means that you create a personal prime directive that no matter how tired you are, you never miss an appointment. There will be times when you will sit there thinking about rescheduling that chemotherapy session today. Just as attitude lets you sleep more than you think you should, it will also get you up and going to continue the treatment. You still might think about not going, but you have to make sure you are not the weak link in your treatment.

51. How long is the recovery period?

Gracy's comment:

At the time I am writing this it has been almost three years since my BMT. I was in the hospital for less than three weeks for the actual procedure. It was two years after BMT that I returned to work. I would say that my BMT and post-BMT period were two years because everything seemed to go right with the procedure itself and the recovery period that followed it. I had no major complications as a result of the BMT. The major part of my recovery period was devoted to allowing my body to build its immune system to normal strength. Once you come home from BMT hospitalization, you continue to be immune compromised. A neighbor, local child, your dog, household mold, and a long list of other contaminants see you as the perfect host. You have to remain relatively isolated from others and think hard about the immune system consequences of anything you do.

I am working today and engaging in all the activities that I want. I feel no physical or mental limitations. I am aware that the BMT process has a tendency to put stress on some organs, such as the lungs and the kidney. I do not smoke cigarettes or drink alcohol anymore. No one had to tell me to discontinue either of these activities. After traveling the BMT road, I have no intention of developing lung cancer or having problems with my kidneys.

I am not cured of leukemia—I have been "in remission" for three years. Remission means that my genes have not told my cells to start going crazy again. This does not mean it cannot happen in the future. Some day I may reach an age that allows me to think I am cured. In a sense, the recovery period will be the rest of my life.

52. Will I have sleeping problems?

Many medications used in the hospital before, during and after the transplant may cause sleeping problems. The chemotherapy used before a transplant very frequently increases anxiety and causes sleep disturbance. The low white blood cell count, or neutropenic, period following transplant may also cause sleep problems. You can control your anxiety and sleep problems with a medication called Ativan, which is frequently used in patients undergoing transplant. Your sleeping problems may persist for some time following transplant and may be made worse by clinical depression, which some patients develop post transplant. Generally, three months post transplant this problem is resolved in most of the patients.

53. When will my immune system recover?

Your immune system will recover much more quickly following an autologous transplant than an allogeneic transplant. The recovery of **blood counts** post transplant occurs within 2 to 4 weeks, but it takes much longer for the immune function to recover. Most

Blood count
a test that measures the number of red blood cells, white blood cells, and platelets in a blood sample.

patients who have had autologous transplants will recover immune function within 6 weeks to 3 months, while it may take 6 to 12 months for the immune system to recover after an allogeneic transplant. Many allogeneic transplant patients (30–50%) will receive immunosuppressive therapy to treat GVHD, which further suppresses the immune system. During the period of suppressed immune system, it is important to avoid crowded places, people with infections, and unknown restaurants. You should discuss these issues with your case manager and transplant physicians.

During the period of suppressed immune system, it is important to avoid crowded places, people with infections, and unknown restaurants.

54. What can I bring to the hospital?

You will be staying in a single room that has limited storage space, so you must be selective about what to bring to the hospital. During your stay in the hospital, your immune system will be compromised, so keeping your room germ free as much as possible is important. Hospital gowns and pants will be provided; however, if you wish, you may bring your own clothing. Try to use gowns that open in the front so that your central venous catheter can be opened easily. You will be required to shower daily and change your clothes after the shower. You must wear stockings or booties while walking in the hospital halls. Your bedding will be changed daily by hospital staff, and laundry will be provided by hospital services. You may want to bring your own pillow (no feather pillows) and a quilt, if they will make you more comfortable. The hospital will provide essential toiletries, but you may wish to bring your own soap, shampoo, lotion, and make-up. If you do this, however, all products must be new and in unopened packages so that they will remain sterile.

The hospital will implement special mouth care, so you do not need to bring a toothbrush or toothpaste. Other items that you may consider bringing are a laptop computer, address book, books, magazines, photos, posters, portable radio/CD player, eyeglasses, and any other items that you may like to have around you while going through this difficult process. Teddy bears are recommended.

Gracy's comment:

The hospital staff provided most of what I needed. What I did bring to the hospital were more personal items, such as a photo of my husband and puppies, a Walkman, hand weights for exercise, a diary, a freshly washed bathrobe (it served as a reminder of what home smelled like), and a Bible.

55. Will I need to wear a mask during hospitalization?

You will not need to wear a mask in your hospital room, which has a special ventilation system as described in Question 40. However, you may need to wear a mask when you leave the room. Also, once you leave the hospital you may need to wear a mask when you come in contact with people who may have a cold or when you walk in large crowds. Still, wearing a mask is not the most important step in preventing infection—hand-washing is. You may be surprised to know this, but wearing a mask does not prevent infection as effectively as hand-washing does. Every transplant room has a hand-washing station next to it, and everyone entering the room must wash his or her hands. This includes staff and visitors.

56. Does my room need to be specially cleaned?

Patients' rooms are designed so that they can be easily cleaned on a daily basis, so that little dust accumulates. Dust can hold various microorganisms, especially fungi, that transplant patients need to avoid at any cost. Rooms are fully cleaned after each patient's stay. Air filters must be changed frequently, depending on how much dust accumulates. A special monitoring system controls the air quality and determines how often the filter should be changed. Floors are usually seamless and easy to clean. Your room will be cleaned daily and as needed. Your windows and your door will remain closed throughout the transplant to prevent pathogenic organisms from getting into your room.

57. Is there a purified water supply in the BMT unit?

Water can be a source of bacterial contamination. Tap water is screened regularly for microorganisms, and many units use special filters for water that is used for washing. Many units also use bottled water for drinking.

58. Can I have visitors?

Most centers will allow visitors to enter the room after thorough hand-washing.

Visits by friends and family are important for your psychological well-being. The frequency of these visits must depend, however, on the stage of your transplantation. Visiting hours and the isolation procedure will vary from center to center. Most centers will allow visitors to enter the room after thorough hand-washing, but some centers will require visitors to wear a special gown. Visitation of young children is at the discretion of your transplant physician. For patients with small children, such visits may be an important issue, and many centers will do all they can to accommodate visits by children. Most centers are relaxing the rules for visits by family members to make the transplant process easier on the patient and family.

59. Will I be able to exercise?

The low energy level that occurs after the transplant prevents many patients from exercising. However, regular exercise is an important part of the recovery process. It has been proven in well-designed studies that people who exercise recover better. Exercise can help counteract problems such as stiff joints, breathing problems, poor appetite, and anxiety. It may be difficult to begin the exercise regime at first, particularly if you have a low platelet count (thrombocytopenia) or active infections. You should start your exercise regimen slowly, beginning with light activity and increasing your level of exercise over time. A good way to initiate exercise may be to take a walk every day or to start physical therapy while staying in the hospital. In transplant units with HEPA-filtered systems, patients are allowed and encouraged to walk in the hallway. Some centers have exercise machines and bicycles that your doctor can prescribe and which you can use frequently. Exercise improves circulation, heart function, muscle strength, sleeping pattern, and overall well-being. It may decrease anxiety and nausea. Exercise is especially important for patients taking steroids long-term, which can weaken muscle and bones. You should pace yourself and exercise only as much as your body allows. The best way to regain strength is through regular exercise suited to your physical strength and ability.

Pace yourself and exercise only as much as your body allows.

60. Will I be able to eat regular foods?

Mucositis

a temporary but painful condition where the lining of the inside of the mouth breaks down, making eating and swallowing difficult.

Intravenous (IV)

entering the body through a vein.

Neutropenic diet

a diet used by people with suppressed immune systems that limits intake of fresh foods in order to lower the possibility of infection.

Many transplant patients will have a poor appetite due to **mucositis** (mouth sores), nausea, and vomiting; some will require **parenteral nutrition** (nutrition, including protein, lipids, glucose, vitamins, and electrolytes, given **intravenously**). Gut decontamination with antibiotics is standard in many transplant centers and may be more important than eating sterile foods.

In many units sterile food is not required; instead, patients are given a low microbial diet called a **neutropenic diet**. This diet excludes fresh fruits and vegetables and raw meats, such as sushi. You may have canned, pasteurized fruits and vegetables. You must follow this diet until your white blood cell counts recover, usually about one month post transplant. There are also other factors that could change the way you eat. Chemotherapy impacts the taste buds in the mouth, and food may taste different for some time after the transplant. Chemotherapy can also cause nausea, vomiting, and indigestion. Avoiding spicy, acidic, or fatty food may help to prevent indigestion. If nausea, vomiting, and indigestion persist, it is important to consult your doctor.

61. Can I smoke cigarettes or drink alcohol?

While you are in the hospital, you cannot smoke. Smoking not only contaminates the purified air of your room (which, of course, you cannot leave), but it's also a fire hazard in areas containing highly flammable chemicals or gases, including the pure oxygen used to help patients with lung problems. It is generally recommended that patients who smoke quit smoking at least two weeks before the transplant. It may help you to use a nicotine transdermal patch (Nicoderm or Habitrol). Patches come in 21 mg, 14 mg, and 7 mg strengths. Generally, the starting dose is 21 mg/day, which should be gradually tapered to 7 mg/day. Quitting smoking will also improve your overall health, making the transplant process easier on your body. It will especially improve your lung function, which can greatly lessen your chance of contracting lung infections as described below.

Quitting smoking will also improve your overall health.

Likewise, you will also not be allowed to drink alcohol, particularly if you are taking chemotherapy medications because it could interact with these drugs. If you regularly drink alcohol and think you might have difficulty with the idea of "going cold turkey" for your transplant, you may wish to speak with your hospital social worker to arrange for help in eliminating alcohol before the transplant.

After you leave the hospital, your risk of lung damage post transplant is much higher, as is your risk of getting lung infections. You should therefore avoid smoking after your transplant. Try to avoid secondhand smoke as well.

You should also avoid any alcohol during the first six months post transplant. Your liver is the main organ processing chemotherapy, so it may not be working at full capacity after the transplant. The liver has a remarkable ability to regenerate, but alcohol harms it, so you should stay away from it altogether. As noted above, do not drink any alcohol if you take medications. The interactions between the alcohol and most medications are unpredictable and may be severe, possibly even life-threatening.

Do not drink any alcohol if you take medications.

62. Will I need special venous access for the procedure?

All patients receiving a bone marrow/stem cell transplant will need a central venous catheter. The catheter is placed into a large vein that leads into your heart and is used to infuse chemotherapy, all medications, intravenous (IV) nutrition (if needed), IV hydration, and blood transfusions. The catheter will remain in place throughout the entire transplant process and, depending on the complications of your transplant and your blood transfusion requirements, several weeks or months post transplant. Before the apheresis a special, large-bore apheresis catheter will be inserted to collect stem cells. The so-called Hickman catheter will be inserted for allogeneic transplant. Both of these catheters can be inserted on an outpatient basis. Your transplant coordinator will teach you how to take care of the catheter, how to keep it clean, flush it, and prevent any infections. You will be told to call the hospital if you have a fever while you have the catheter. Sometimes, when the catheter gets clotted or infected it needs to be removed and replaced.

Gracy's comment:

I had not just one but two types of catheters put in my chest. The first one was called Port-o-cath. A trauma surgeon attached it to a main vein under my skin. The port is invisible once the site heals and provides convenient access for chemotherapy treatment. This catheter was inserted on the right side of my chest. It was invisible because a layer of my skin grew over it. When medical staff wanted to use it they would use a needle to poke through the skin and access the port. It is worth mentioning that some cancer drugs delay the body's healing function. In my case, my catheter surgical site took six months to heal. I called this type of catheter an internal catheter because it could stay in my body for years and only needed to be flushed (to prevent clotting) every six weeks. This catheter can only be removed through surgery once it is no longer needed.

In preparation for any unexpected emergency and to provide access for delivering multiple medications to my body simultaneously, my doctor felt it necessary to have an additional catheter. The second catheter was called a Hickman catheter. A surgeon inserted this catheter on the left side of my chest. The hole was a little larger than the end of a ballpoint pen. I called this type of catheter an external catheter because it is visible and requires weekly flushing, and its life cycle is not as long as that of the internal catheter.

63. How do I care for my catheter?

The exit site of your catheter must be cleaned frequently to prevent infection. The catheter goes directly into your bloodstream, so keeping it clean is essential in preventing bacterial infections. While you are in the hospital, your catheter will be cleaned with alcohol and betadine, and the site will be covered with sterile gauze. You should cover the exit site with a plastic bag while you shower to avoid damaging it with moisture. Dressings must be changed frequently, every 1 to 2 days. Your physician or a nurse will inspect the site daily while you are in the hospital. It is important that you notify the case manager immediately if you notice redness or pus around the site of the catheter. Signs of infection include pain, redness, tenderness when touched, oozing, and fever. Your catheter may have several separate lines, which need to be clamped properly. Your nurse will give you detailed instruction on how to clamp your catheter properly.

Gracy's comment:

Doctors and nurses can give you detailed instructions on how to care for your catheter, but you are the one who lives with it and has to sleep with it. I was overwhelmed and paranoid when the catheter was first put in. I was afraid that germs could get through the tube at any time and infect my body. At first I was also very uncomfortable having the catheter on my body and having to watch out for it like an additional body part.

I overcame my fear of infection by taking time to learn. I learned how to inspect for infection, how to flush it when necessary, how to tape off the site before taking a shower, and so on. Overcoming the fear really helped me when I was discharged and went home with the catheter still embedded in my chest.

Time also allowed me to adjust to the catheter as an additional body part. In time, having the catheter is as natural as having an arm. Being a woman, the ability to tuck the tube attached to the catheter into my bra made my life much easier.

YOUR HEALTHCARE TEAM

64. Who is involved in my healthcare team?

The healthcare team involved in your transplant consists of your physicians, a BMT transplant representative, a case manager, an apheresis nurse, a dietitian, a pharmacist, a physical therapist, in-patient nurses, a social worker, and the Hospital Unit Service Coordinator (HUSC). They all work together and help each other so that your transplant proceeds as smoothly and efficiently as possible. Two attending physicians will be involved: the primary attending physician, who will be involved in all aspects of your care, and the inpatient attending physician, who will be involved in your inpatient care on a daily basis. These two physicians work together very closely, and they discuss the progress of your transplant with all of your physicians at least weekly. At times, depending on schedules, your primary physician and inpatient attending physician are the same person. Sometimes fellows—that is, physicians in training—are involved; they closely report to the attending physician.

A specific case manager will be assigned to you and will work very closely with you on all aspects of your transplant: pre-transplant work-up, transplant procedure, and post-transplant follow up. He or she will be the first one to answer your phone calls, educate you on your pre-transplant work-up and post-transplant issues, follow up on your lab results, and facilitate communication with the physician. The social worker will meet with you for pre-transplant evaluation and will evaluate all the social and psychological needs that you may have, as well the level of support you will be able to obtain. He or she will help you to obtain social support, insurance changes, or disability leave from work. The social worker will visit you during your hospital stay, and you should feel free to voice any concerns you may have. The nurses on the inpatient transplant unit are very highly qualified and will also work closely with you so that this difficult process can proceed smoothly. They are highly competent and compassionate individuals who are very devoted to their patients. At times it may be possible for you to have a primary nurse, who will be assigned to you on most of the shifts.

There are often two primary medical team members involved throughout the entire BMT procedure. If you have a form of cancer, one may be your primary **oncologist**, who is the doctor treating your cancer and likely the one who initiated your referral for transplantation. For other, non-cancer blood diseases, this role is probably played by a **hematologist**, a doctor specializing in

Oncologist

a physician who specializes in cancer treatment.

Hematologist

a specialist who sees and treats patients with malignancies (and other diseases) of the blood.

blood diseases. The other doctor is the transplant physician, who coordinates everything initiated by the primary oncologist/hematologist as well as all BMT-related matters not directly involving the primary oncologist/hematologist. The primary doctor provides "doctor's orders" and the transplant coordinator makes sure that those orders are carried out. For example, your primary oncologist authorizes blood products for your use, orders tests, and answers queries from your health maintenance organization (HMO). The transplant coordinator makes sure the blood products are obtained and given to you as directed and that the tests are performed and the results delivered to the primary oncologist, and interacts directly with the representatives of your HMO. In effect, the transplant coordinator is the source of all your information in planning for everything that you must do before, during, and after the BMT procedure.

Gracy's comment:

My BMT could not have been as successful as it was without a seamless, collective effort from a caring social worker who would listen to me cry; a friendly kitchen worker who would bring my meals to my hospital bed; an understanding nurse who came to check my temperature in the middle of the night; and a friendly nurse assistant who would chat with me while making my bed. There were countless people involved in my care. All of them did their part to make my transplant procedure go smoothly.

65. Is the nursing staff specially trained in BMT units?

Nursing staff employed on the BMT unit must be specially trained. The nurse/patient ratio may vary from 1:1 for complicated problems to 1:3 or even 1:4 for patients whose cases are not complicated. Nurses must be familiar with the application and complications of high dose chemotherapy. They must be able to recognize unstable patients and patients with acute GVHD. In many BMT units, standard orders for fever ("fever protocol"), administration of blood products ("transfusion protocol"), chemotherapy, and intravenous hydration are used. These standard orders facilitate the care of these patients with complicated needs and avoid confusion that may occur among rotating physicians or fellows.

66. *What are nurse staff ratios, and why are they important?*

Nurse staffing ratios are the number of nurses in a particular hospital that cover a given number of patients. The hospital administration tries to reach a fair balance between quality of care and cost of care. Quality of care is what affects you the most! Cost of care, while important, should not prevent you from getting what you need.

The ideal situation is to have enough nurses available. When this is the case, the nursing staff can devote their time to making sure that your experience in the hospital is a positive one. The nurse can address your emotional concerns as well as your physical needs. Nurse training focuses on the emotional well being of the patient as well as health problems. Nurses can use all the skills they have developed if given the opportunity—and the time.

When nurses don't have the time to use their skills and training, some things are going to slip. No matter how devoted nurses are to their profession and their patients, they are also human. They can only do so much at one time and, if overworked, they can become tired and irritable.

If you have a serious problem, such as pain or unusual symptoms, a nurse should come immediately.

When you panic at two o'clock in the morning and you press the help button next to your bed, the time you spend waiting can seem like an eternity. At times it can be so reassuring to talk to a nurse about a concern you have without having her look at her watch or turn her head toward the door because she has a thousand other things she should be doing. But keep in mind that you're not the only patient there and not the nurse's only responsibility. If no one responds quickly when you just want to talk, don't get upset; the nurses may be coping with other seriously ill patients' health needs, which surely take priority. However, if you have a serious problem, such as pain or unusual symptoms, a nurse *should* come immediately, and you have the right to complain if you are left waiting for long stretches of time when you need care.

PART FOUR

The BMT Procedure

What is the BMT conditioning regimen?

What are the side effects of conditioning chemotherapy?

What are the immediate complications of the conditioning regimen?

More . . .

Preparing You for Transplant

67. What is the BMT conditioning regimen?

The next stage of treatment after the stem cell collection is conditioning regimen (also called the preparative regimen). It involves several days of chemotherapy with or without irradiation. The type and amount of chemotherapy you receive depends on your disease, type of transplant, and your overall condition. The goals of the conditioning regimen are to destroy the diseased cells in your body, create space in your bone marrow for the new cells, and suppress your immune system to reduce the risk of rejection. The chemotherapy is often given through a central line over several days. Some people experience nausea and vomiting during the chemotherapy, but the newest premedication regimens can reduce these side effects in many patients. The radiation therapy treatment, if you need it, is painless and may be given before or after the chemotherapy. The effects of conditioning therapy range from mild to severe. The common side effects of conditioning therapy are nausea, vomiting, diarrhea, hair loss, fatigue, loss of appetite, and mouth sores. Most people develop only some of these side effects. The conditioning therapy may also irritate your bladder and cause blood to appear in your urine; you should report this symptom so that it can be treated with blood irrigation through a Foley catheter.

Gracy's comment:

I thought that prior chemotherapy had sucked all the energy that was left in me. Then I discovered that I had to undergo a conditioning regimen that consisted of high-dose chemotherapy and a total body irradiation (TBI). The conditioning regimen really began to take a toll on my body and I was nauseated. But do you know what? This is when your attitude really comes in handy. Whenever I had an urge to vomit, I just said "No!" So remember, just say no, and you will be amazed at how your body responds.

68. What are the side effects of conditioning chemotherapy?

You may have minimal, moderate, or severe side effects of high-dose chemotherapy. Shortly after chemotherapy you may experience nausea, vomiting, diarrhea, and irregular heartbeat. About 1 to 2 weeks following the treatment, you may experience nausea, vomiting, liver damage, hair loss, mouth and throat sores, anemia, and low platelet counts. It is also possible that, over the long term, you may experience infertility and cataracts. It is common for the reproductive organs to be damaged, which results in infertility. Your age, sex, stage of disease, and the intensity of your conditioning regimen can all affect the likelihood of infertility. About 20% of patients develop cataracts, but doctors can remove them surgically in an outpatient setting once you have recovered from your transplant. You will learn more about the side effects of chemotherapy in your pre-transplant sessions. Very few patients have severe side effects.

Very few patients have severe side effects.

Gracy's comment:

I was able to endure the fear of potential side effects and the actual short-term side effects by exercising a positive attitude. I told myself that my hair could grow back, a damaged liver can regenerate, the mouth sores and the sore throat would heal. It is important to remember that in most cases side effects are only temporary and they are part of your recovery.

While I did not develop cataracts, my reproductive organs and ovarian functions were destroyed. I now take a supplement that replenishes estrogen to protect myself from developing osteoporosis.

69. What are the immediate complications of the conditioning regimen?

High-dose chemotherapy can suppress your blood cell counts, which can cause infections and a greater chance of bleeding. You can prevent these problems by taking prophylactic antibiotics and having a transfusion of platelets. Patients who have a low white blood count and develop fever must submit a blood culture and take broad-spectrum antibiotics. Some patients who have had chemotherapy before or are older may experience multi-organ failure. The most common complication, however, involves the liver and is called **vaso-occlusive disease** of the liver (VOD; see Question 76). Patients with high risk for VOD will take Lovenox (long-acting heparin) during the transplant for prophylaxis (prevention). One of the most common side effects of the pre-transplant conditioning is **mucositis**, which is the breakdown of the moist lining, or mucosa, in the mouth and gastrointestinal system. This leads to the formation of small ulcers (sores). Doctors can treat mucositis with supportive measures, pain control, and intravenous nutrition. You may also notice skin changes, such as hyperpigmentation (darkened skin) and nail changes.

Vaso-occlusive disease (VOD)

a sometimes fatal condition that can lead to liver failure; requires rapid medical intervention.

70. What kind of chemotherapy agents are used for stem cell therapy?

Doctors use different conditioning regimens for autologous and allogeneic stem cell transplant. One of the most common conditioning regimens for stem cell transplant, especially with patients who have acute leukemia or high-risk lymphoma, is Cy/TBI (cyclophosphamide combined with total body irradiation). Another common regimen for chronic myelogenous leukemia (CML) is Bu/CY (busulfan and cyclophosphamide). Busulfan works well against leukemia and has fewer side effects than TBI, but it can cause vaso-occlusive diseases of the liver (VOD) in some patients (see Question 76). Patients with diseases such as lupus erythematosus (SLE) will receive a high dose of cyclophosphamide with or without anti-thymocyte globulin (ATG).

Patients who have had solid organ transplant will receive different combinations of chemotherapeutic agents, sometimes composed of four to six different agents to enhance the anti-tumor activity.

Mini-allogeneic transplant patients receive either low-dose irradiation (400 cGy) in combination with fludarabine ("Seattle approach"), or a combination of cyclophosphamide and fludarabine ("MD Anderson approach"). There are at least 10, if not more, different regimens for mini-allogeneic transplant, which vary with different transplant centers.

71. What is total body irradiation (TBI)?

Conditioning regimens for leukemia frequently use irradiation to help suppress the patient's immune system. Unlike radiation treatments for tumors, this radiation is given to your entire body rather than just the portion where cancer is growing—hence the name, total body irradiation (TBI). It is typically given in several sessions, which are called fractionated TBI or hyper-fractionated TBI. Each session lasts from 15 to

45 minutes; although the radiation itself is painless, sometimes patients must spend long periods in an awkward position, which can be uncomfortable. Following the irradiation patients may experience weakness, low energy, nausea, and mouth sores. TBI penetrates the brain well and can profoundly suppress the immune system.

Gracy's comment:

I had read of all the horrible side effects of total body irradiation (stunted growth, memory problems, inability to concentrate, and so on). I wished God would spare me from this procedure. But my doctor told me that she did not want to see any remnants of diseased cells remaining in my body. They could hide in my central nervous system during the conditioning regimen and come back and haunt me after the transplant. Once again, left with no choice, I confronted my fear and accepted the TBI treatment.

During each TBI session I sat on a leather seat similar to the mechanical bull that people ride in bars. Its height was adjusted to my height so I could put my weight on it when I got tired. A harness was attached to my upper body and secured by an overhead support. This equipment was needed to keep me still while the x-ray machine was irradiating my body. I felt like I was standing in the transport room of the Starship Enterprise and was about to dematerialize for transport through space. I had plenty of time to think of these things because the TBI took 45 minutes to complete. My heart and lungs were the only parts of my body that were not irradiated. At the end of each session I honestly didn't know if I was on earth or in space. My mental and physical state was so poor that I did not know if I was coming or going. It is extremely important to have someone accompany you to each session and be there for you when it is time to go home. ***Do not even think about driving yourself home!***

TBI is the jumping off point. It is similar to the moment before someone jumps from a plane with his or her parachute. TBI destroys your immune system. From this point on you are vulnerable to bacterial and viral infections from everything around you. Not only that, but you are also vulnerable to various infections from within your own body. This is very similar to what happens to people who have full-blown AIDS. They can get sick and die from a common cold or bacteria that are normally in your stomach and kept in check by your immune system. The medical people call this dangerously low immune protection, or neutropenia.

It is extremely important to have someone accompany you to each session and be there for you when it is time to go home.

72. What are the side effects of total body irradiation?

Total body irradiation (TBI) is a necessary part of the transplant process because it kills the diseased cells in preparation for infusion of healthy stem cells. However, the radiation also affects healthy cells in the body quite dramatically and can be difficult for the patient. The side effects of TBI are quite a daunting list: nausea and vomiting, diarrhea, fever, parotitis (inflammation of the gland next to the ear; when the inflammation occurs, you may look like you have the mumps), skin rash, mucositis, interstitial pneumonitis, sterility, thyroid dysfunction, impairment of growth and development, and secondary malignancies—cancers that start because of the radiation, unrelated to the disease you currently have.

All patients will have nausea and vomiting toward the end of the irradiation schedule. Vomiting may be quite severe in the beginning, and should go away 3 to 4 days after irradiation. The good news is that your doctor can treat these symptoms using anti-emetic medications such as ondansetrone or compazine. If you experience nausea and vomiting, you should immediately tell your doctor or nurse. Some patients will experience parotitis (inflammation of the parotid gland located in front of the ear) with jaw pain that will go away in 2 to 3 days. A short course of steroids is effective in such cases. A few days after irradiation, you may get a skin rash, which could intensify ("radiation recall") if you are receiving chemotherapy at the same time.

Other side effects related to TBI aren't as obvious, and they may appear later. For example, most children who receive TBI will have decreased growth rates. Girls may have an average of 4.0 cm growth decrease, and boys may have a 4.5 cm growth decrease two years post transplant. Also, most (40–55%) patients develop thyroid dysfunction post TBI. The most common problem is compensated hypothyroidism (decreased thyroid function). The symptoms associated with hypothyroidism are increased fatigue, sleepiness, excessive weight gain, dry and thinning hair, dry skin, and feelings of coldness. Patients with hypothyroidism may take thyroid hormone tablets (replacement therapy). Some patients develop cataracts (see Question 73), and some doctors believe that the radiation causes other cancers (see Question 74).

Despite these serious side effects, however, TBI is an important part of the conditioning regimens for aggressive cancers. Remember, the side effects described above are *possible*, not certain, so TBI may be a better bet than letting your original disease take its course.

73. Could I develop cataracts after TBI?

TBI regimens can cause cataracts. Cataracts are more severe in patients who receive a single dose of radiation therapy than in those who get fractionated treatment—that is, radiation therapy in which only a small portion of the total dose is given in one session, so that the patient must come for a number of sessions to get the full dose. The smallest dose known to cause cataracts in humans is 200 cGy in a single fraction and 400–550 cGy in multiple doses. There is a big difference in the rate of cataract development depending on what kind of radiation is given: 80% of patients who receive TIB of more than 200 cGy develop cataracts, but this rate can be lowered to less than 20% if the patients receive fractionated treatment. Cataracts may not appear immediately after treatment; it can take from 6 months to 3 or 4 years for cataracts to form. About 20 to 50% of patients who receive TBI will eventually need surgery to remove cataracts.

Cataracts also occur in patients who get radiation that is not TBI, but it is much less common. About 18% of patients with aplastic anemia who receive non-TBI based regimens get cataracts. Steroids and GVHD can also cause cataracts.

74. Does TBI cause secondary cancers?

Doctors don't know whether TBI causes secondary cancers. Different reports provide different numbers, but one large tumor registry reported that 127 of 9,880 patients developed secondary cancers. One of the largest transplant centers in the world, Fred Hutchinson Cancer Center in Seattle, reported that patients are 3.9 times more likely to develop a second cancer after TBI. It is therefore very important for you to have early cancer screenings, such as mammography, pelvic exams, and PAP smears for women, prostate exams for men, and colorectal and skin screening for all patients. You should also avoid tobacco and excessive alcohol after your transplant.

75. What is graft failure?

Graft failure

rejection of transplanted cells by the recipient. Also called graft rejection.

"Graft" is simply another word for your transplanted cells. **Graft failure**, also called **graft rejection,** occurs when your body rejects transplanted stem cells and your blood cell counts do not recover properly. Graft rejection only happens in allogeneic transplants, and then only if enough T-cells survive conditioning (pre-transplant chemotherapy) to reject the graft. You have a greater risk of graft rejection if your transplant was from a matched unrelated donor than if it was from an HLA-identical sibling. This is because when the cells are HLA-matched, your immune system is fooled into thinking that the donated cells belong to you—and the closer the match, the more likely it is that your immune system will be tricked into accepting the new cells. About 5 to 20% of patients who receive bone marrow from unrelated donors experience graft failure. Patients who receive **T-cell depleted transplants** (transplants using bone marrow that has been subjected to a procedure that removes the lymphocytes) have the highest chance of graft failure. Sometimes a back-up supply of stem cells is kept in the lab so your team can re-infuse them in case you experience graft failure.

T-cell depleted transplant

a transplant in which lymphocytes are removed from the donated bone marrow prior to transplantation.

Your risk of graft failure also depends on the previous condition of your bone marrow, your disease type, the type of transplant you are having, and the number of stem cells infused. It also depends on whether or not T lymphocytes were infused because lymphocytes help to achieve **engraftment**. Sometimes stem cells do not grow well and simply fail to engraft, but on rare occasions graft failure may also be caused by certain infections or medications. If this happens, your doctors will try to re-infuse the cells.

Engraftment
the process by which a transplant patient's body accepts the donor's cells and incorporates them into normal bodily functions.

76. What is VOD?

VOD stands for vaso-occlusive disease of the liver, which is a common complication of allogeneic stem cell transplants when patients have been heavily pre-treated with chemotherapy and/or radiation therapy (See Questions 67–69 and 71–74). It happens when small blood vessels in the liver become damaged and are blocked by clotting factors. This blockage causes fluid retention and leakage of fluids due to the decrease in the level of blood **albumin**. Albumin, a protein produced in the liver that is released into the bloodstream, helps to maintain fluids inside this space. When the damaged liver cannot produce enough albumin to stop this fluid retention and leakage, it leads to further problems: clotting is activated in the liver, the liver swells, and bilirubin (a product of the blood pigment processed in the liver) increases in the blood. Sometimes this process causes with kidney failure and is called hepato-renal syndrome.

Albumin
a protein produced in the liver that helps retain fluid in the liver.

VOD can be mild, moderate, or severe. Most patients who have a mild form will survive, and the treatment is mainly supportive. On the other hand, patients who have a severe form need intensive therapy with anti-coagulating agents, such as t-PA, and some patients will die. In many heavily pretreated patients, Lovenox (long-acting heparin) is instituted. Heparin is a chemical that prevents formation of blood clots. Patients can take it to prevent VOD as well as to treat it.

77. What is CMV infection?

CMV

cytomegalovirus; a virus that can cause pneumonia, hepatitis, and gastrointestinal illness.

CMV stands for **cytomegalovirus**. CMV is similar to the herpes virus, but it is much more dangerous, particularly to people with poor immune systems. It can cause pneumonia, inflammation of the liver, and gastrointestinal diseases. In very immunocompromised patients it can cause inflammation of the retina in the eye, which can lead to blindness. This is, however, a rare occurrence. CMV is a common virus, and many people have been exposed to it and have it living inactively in their bodies. However, when a patient is immunocompromised, this virus can become active again and cause a disease. A blood test may be able to find this early. If your doctor learns that you have CMV, you can take a medication called gancyclovir to help control it. It is common to test patients who undergo allogeneic stem cell transplant weekly for CMV. Early treatment can prevent you from developing of severe disease, including some diseases that often caused death in the past (most commonly pneumonia).

78. What is done to prevent or control infections?

The most important rule for preventing infections is hand-washing.

All institutions have different infection prevention guidelines, but most transplant centers have the same basic rules. It is important to follow these guidelines to prevent infections in transplant units. The most important rule is hand-washing. This rule applies to nurses and doctors as well as to all visitors. The air quality in the unit is measured by counting the air particles and by measuring how much and what kinds of bacteria and fungi are in the air. The hospital does cultures of skin, mucous membranes, stool, and urine samples on a regular basis. Many patients receive gut decontamination and aggressive antibiotic treatment. Despite all these measures, infections such as human herpesvirus 6 (HHV–6), adenovirus, BK virus, and invasive Aspergillus are still a problem in many transplant units. It is important that you be very conscientious about washing your own hands regularly and monitoring your visitors to make sure that they follow the rules.

79. Will I become sterile?

Many patients undergoing stem cell therapy are young. If you are a woman of childbearing age or a man who wants children in the future, your doctor will advise you before therapy that you may become permanently sterile. If you want to have children in the future, you should discuss arrangements for sperm or oocyte (egg) banking with your doctor before your treatment begins. This process may take several weeks or months, so you should discuss it as early as posslible in the transplant process.

You may become permanently sterile.

The Main Event

80. How is bone marrow transported to a transplant center?

Your donor's bone marrow will be collected into a standard blood transfer bag (600–2,000 mL volume). The bag will be labeled with your name and the donor's name (when the donor is related) or identifying number (when your donor is unrelated), and a courier will carry it from the operating room to a processing laboratory of a transplant center. If the bone marrow is from an unrelated donor, it will be transported on wet ice or in an insulated container, and must arrive at the transplant center within 24 hours of when it was harvested. Marrows are collected and transported worldwide, so this process can happen any time of day. Therefore, the receiving laboratory may need to have people working 24 hours a day. If nothing must be done with the bone marrow, it may be infused almost immediately after it arrives; if the bone marrow needs to be processed one way or another, you may not receive the infusion for 3 to 6 hours.

81. What happens during the transplant procedure itself?

The day of stem cell transplant is an exciting day for many patients, and they think of it as a "birthday" or a new beginning in life. The procedure is surprisingly simple: a bag or several bags of bone marrow or peripheral blood stem cells is infused over several hours through a central line, just like any other blood product or medication. Once the stem cells enter your bloodstream, they move through your body with your blood. Within several days, they "home" to the spaces in your bone marrow, where they settle and grow. It will take 1 to 2 weeks before new cells show up in your blood in the form of recovering white blood cells (that is, new white blood cells growing from the implanted stem cells). The new red blood cells usually show up next, and platelets last. In the meantime, you will be supported with the blood and platelet transfusions as required.

Gracy's comment:

August 23rd, 1999, Day 0, the nurse wheeled several steel cases into my room. The stem cells were previously frozen in plastic bags and stored in the steel cases. I watched the nurse thawing plastic bags right in front of my eyes. It took 5 to 10 minutes for her to thaw each bag in a tray of warm water. The thawing process made the stem cells come alive, and they had to be infused into my body within 20 minutes. A bag of stem cells looks similar to a unit of blood. Each bag was hung from an intravenous (IV) tube, which was attached to a catheter on my chest. As the stem cells were entering my body, so was the chemical that was used to preserve the stem cell. The chemical created a garlicky taste and filled my lungs as if I was holding a chest full of cigarette smoke. This discomfort lasted only a few minutes.

82. What is engraftment, and when does it occur?

Engraftment will happen within 1 to 3 weeks after your transplant (counted from the day the stem cells were infused), when the newly infused cells begin to grow in your bone marrow. Engraftment usually occurs earlier with peripheral stem cell transplant than when the stem cells are obtained from the bone marrow. When the stem cells are obtained from the bone marrow, engraftment will usually take 2 to 4 weeks. Throughout this period, your doctors will monitor your blood count carefully for signs of engraftment. They will pay particular attention to your neutrophil count, which is also called your absolute neutrophil count (ANC). Neutrophil are important white blood cells that fight infection. Therefore, your doctors will watch you closely during the period called neutropenia, when the white blood cell count is low. They will give you antibiotics if you develop a fever.

Gracy's comment:

When I first moved into my hospital room I saw a blackboard hanging on the wall. I could not imagine what the blackboard could be for. As it turned out, this blackboard is where my "engraftment" success was tracked over time. Following the stem cell infusion, the nursing staff took my blood and sent it to the lab for testing every day for signs that the engraftment was taking place. This status was tracked on the blackboard by daily counts of my red blood cells, white blood cells, and platelets.

I could clearly see that on Day 0 (the day I was infused with stem cells), the blackboard did not show a trace of a living white cell, red cell, or platelet. My body was totally defenseless against any form of infection because I had no immune system. I felt so weak that I thought I could close my eyes, go to sleep, and never wake up again. My cell count remained at 0 for the first 7 days. On the 8th day, a miracle happened. The columns on the blackboard started to show numbers. The new stem cells had found a home inside my bones and had started to manufacture healthy cells. It was the most exciting and amazing experience in the world to see how the cells multiplied over time. They went from 40 to 100 to 1000 in a very short time. The numbers that the nurse wrote on the blackboard became a strong physical symbol of how successfully the procedure was taking. Brenda's new cells had grafted inside my bones and were now living in my body.

83. What is a low microbial diet?

All transplant patients are on this diet starting on the day of admission to the hospital. Autologous transplant patients may resume a regular diet after their transplant. However, patients who have had an allogeneic transplant cannot resume a regular diet until after they recover their blood counts and immune function. The general rules for a low microbial diet are: all foods must be cooked well to 170–180 degrees Fahrenheit, all cold foods must be served packed in a plastic wrap, and there must be strict adherence to all dietary and sanitary guidelines. The low microbial diet meets the Recommended Dietary Allowances.

84. What is total parenteral nutrition (TPN)?

If you cannot maintain proper nutrition by mouth, you will be given **total parenteral nutrition** (TPN). Conditioning radiation and chemotherapy often damage the mucosa of the mouth, a condition called mucositis. This can make it difficult to eat. TPN provides protein, carbohydrates, fats, vitamins, and minerals for essential nutrition. You will receive TPN intravenously over 12 to 24 hours. You may eat while receiving TPN, and it will be discontinued when you demonstrate that you can eat and maintain proper nutrition.

Total parenteral nutrition
nutrition supplied intravenously instead of by mouth.

85. What is the hospital routine during transplant?

You will probably be in the hospital a long time during your transplant, usually 2 weeks up to 3 months. It is possible that you will need to stay longer if you develop unusual complications. Most of the patients who receive autologous transplant will be released from the hospital within two weeks. The patients who have allogeneic transplant will leave the hospital some time between 1 to 3 months. While you are in the hospital, you will have a regular routine. You will start your morning with a shower, your bedding will be changed, and your doctors will examine you and discuss your progress with you. Either before or after the medical rounds, you will take all of your medications. After the rounds, you may need to undergo some procedures such as x-rays, CT scans, or nutrition and social consult. You will eat meals at regular times through the day, usually at 8, 12, and 6, and you will get extra snacks in the afternoon. You may request special dishes according to your needs. If you cannot eat enough food to sustain your nutrition, you may receive total parenteral nutrition (TPN) by vein. Throughout the day, your fluid balance, vital signs, and general condition will be assessed. In the afternoon, you may take a walk (usually with a mask), visit with friends or family, and exercise. An afternoon nap is highly recommended, since your energy level during this time may be quite low. You will have a nurse assigned to you overnight, and you can request sleeping pills if you have problems sleeping.

PART FIVE

Post Transplant

What is discharge planning?

What do I need to do before going home?

What about food? Do I need to take any special precautions post transplant?

More . . .

86. What is discharge planning?

Discharge planning

the process of preparing a transplant patient to leave the hospital into a controlled, clean, safe environment where the patient has less likelihood of getting an infection post transplant.

Discharge planning from the hospital starts on the day you are admitted. Most patients will be discharged from the hospital at 2 to 4 weeks post transplant. The discharge process may be overwhelming and intimidating because you need to absorb so much information. That is why discharge education begins early, so everything can be prepared and explained to you in advance. This will include information such as how to clean your home properly, how to prepare food, how to handle animals and pets, how to advance physical activity, what to do in case of fever, how to relate to the sun, and so on. Many centers will have a booklet describing these issues in detail.

Gracy's comment:

After being watched around the clock for complications for nearly two weeks, I looked to doctors, nurses, and medical devices for protection and continuation of my healthy recovery. Thoughts of hospital discharge gave me mixed feelings. On one hand, I was excited to reunite with my loved ones, and on the other hand, I was terrified of leaving the protective confines of the hospital as well as all the doctors and nurses who were around in case something happened to me.

Taking small steps at a time and following the discharge instructions to the letter, I slowly began to embrace the new life without a hospital room, doctors, 24-hour on-call nurses and medical devices.

87. What do I need to do before going home?

Because of your compromised immune status post transplant, your home must be thoroughly cleaned before you can be discharged from the hospital. The guidelines for cleanliness vary depending on the type of transplant you had and how immunosuppressed you are. The amount of dust, mold, and fungus in the house should be kept to an absolute minimum, as these can transmit infection and disease. Your bathrooms and kitchen should be cleaned thoroughly and you should replace your sponges frequently. The refrigerator should be cleaned before you store food. You should use a cleaner with anti-bacterial disinfectant properties, such as Lysol and bleach. You should also dust with a damp cloth.

88. What about food? Do I need to take any special precautions post transplant?

You will have a greater chance of developing food-related infections until your immune system fully recovers. Before you leave the hospital, you will learn how to follow food safety guidelines. The general recommended rules are:

1. Do not use any food products that are out of date.
2. Do not buy or use any bulging or damaged cans.
3. Make sure frozen foods are solid and refrigerated foods are cold.
4. Do not use cracked eggs.
5. Store and refrigerate groceries promptly after shopping.
6. Do not buy bulk foods from self-service bins.

Food Preparation

Clean cutting boards with a solution of 10 parts water mixed with 1 part bleach. Use separate cutting boards for cooked foods and raw foods. Wash the can opener and tops of cans before you use them. Wash, rinse, and peel fruits and vegetables thoroughly before eating them. Cool and thaw foods inside the refrigerator. Cook all meats well. Do not eat uncooked eggs. Do not eat perishable foods that have been left outside the refrigerator for more than an hour. Do not eat foods that have been stored in the refrigerator for more than three days.

Foods to Avoid

Do not eat free food samples and foods from street vendors. Do not eat or drink soft-serve ice cream, milk shakes, raw eggs, unpasteurized honey and milk, unroasted nuts, aged and moldy cheeses, well water, unrefrigerated cream, mayonnaise-based foods, sushi, or raw fish. Call your doctor to ask what food should be avoided if you have any questions.

89. Will my contacts with other people be restricted after the transplant?

You will have to restrict contact with other people for several months following your transplant.

You will have to restrict contact with other people for several months following your transplant. You must restrict hugging or touching to a few special people with whom you have frequent contact. You must avoid crowded places, such as movie theaters and shopping centers, for at least three months post transplant. You should avoid kindergarten or school settings, since children are more likely to carry infectious diseases than adults. It is best to avoid babies or children who have been vaccinated with live vaccines. If someone living with you is sick, check with your doctor about how you should limit contact with that person. If you choose to eat at restaurants, make sure that it has a reputation for cleanliness and fresh food. Do not hesitate to ask when foods were prepared. Many restaurants will accommodate you.

90. Can I keep pets or plants at home?

You should avoid keeping fresh plants and flowers in your home after your transplant. Different organisms can grow in dirt, water, and plants and cause infection. In general, you should avoid handling plants during the first few months following your transplant. For the same reason, you should avoid contact with soil, lawn waste, and compost. You must limit your contact with animals and household pets during the first 100 days post transplant. During this time, you should not clean up after your pets or touch any human or animal excrement. Specifically, try to avoid litter boxes and birdcages.

91. How can home care help me?

During the BMT procedure, you will be surrounded by professional nursing staff who will provide a carefree environment while meeting your medical needs. But what happens when you are discharged from the hospital? Who will flush your catheters so that blood won't clot? Who will look for signs of infection around your catheters? Who will give you a shot when you need one? Who will perform other medical functions for you? The answer is either you or a home-care professional. If you don't think you are capable of following instructions to care for yourself after leaving the hospital, we strongly recommend that you subscribe to a home-care service. Home-care nurses are specially trained, chemotherapy certified, and bone marrow/stem cell qualified registered nurses who provide teaching, reinforcement, and care at home. Your homecare nurse can communicate with the rest of your care team to manage your home care. A good health plan will cover the cost of home-care service until you are well enough to be on your own.

92. What about construction sites, exposure to sun, and the use of swimming pools post transplant?

Construction Sites

Construction sites are full of dust that may contain fungus and other organisms. You should avoid construction sites post transplant. Roll up the windows when you drive, and make sure your vent or air conditioning is switched to the recirculating feature so that outside air does not come into your car. Try to go around the block when you see a construction site in your neighborhood; if you cannot avoid the site, cover your nose and mouth with a handkerchief and wash thoroughly once you get indoors.

Exposure to Sun

Chemotherapy and radiation used during transplantation may increase your sensitivity to the sun, and therefore you should avoid the sun as much as possible. Sun may make the graft-versus-host disease worse. During your first year post transplant, use sunscreen with a sun protection factor (SPF) of 25 or greater when you go outdoors. On sunny days, wear protective clothing such as hats, sunglasses, and long-sleeved shirts for at least a year post transplant.

Swimming Pools

You should avoid swimming in public lakes or pools until your immune system is fully reconstituted. If you have had an autologous transplant, this will take several months. If you have had an allogeneic transplant, in which the stem cells came from an unrelated donor, you must avoid swimming pools for at least a year. Check with your physician before swimming again.

93. Do I need to make any nutritional adjustments post transplant?

After the transplant, your body will require special nutrients to regain its strength and function. Your nutritional requirements will vary depending on your type of transplant, your general condition, the medications you are taking, and your lifestyle. You may need to talk to a nutritionist about your nutrition requirements. These services are available in most transplant centers. You may be nauseated and find it difficult to eat and drink post transplant. If you do, a good and proven strategy is to eat small portions frequently throughout the day, instead of three large meals. You may take vitamins and minerals in addition to your regular meals. You may also need to drink more fluids to help your digestive system work better. Many people experience dehydration soon after their transplant. You may need intravenous infusions if your dehydration cannot be treated orally.

Your body will require special nutrients to regain its strength and function.

94. Will there be any physical changes related to the transplant process?

Your body will undergo many changes related to your transplant. These changes will affect how you look and feel, your energy level, the functioning of different organs, and your general perception of life. You will probably lose your hair, but it will grow back and usually looks better afterwards. Your skin may be slightly hyperpigmented, but this should get better over time.

Your sexual drive may be affected. You may not be able to run as you had before. Your appetite and taste may change, since your taste buds will be affected by the chemotherapy and change your perception of taste. This change is temporary. Your sleeping pattern may change as well. Many changes will resolve with time, usually within the first year post transplant.

Many changes will resolve with time.

95. What about sexual activity?

In general, sexual activity is safe, as long as you maintain good hygiene and have no sexually transmissible diseases. You may want to talk to a member of your transplant team to find out whether there are any specific reasons for you not to participate in sexual activity. Some transplant centers advise against oral-genital sex as long as the immune system is immunocompromised. Anal sex should be avoided until your platelet count has recovered to the level of 35,000 or higher. The use of condoms is generally recommended, although in a monogamous relationship in which there is no evidence of sexually transmittable diseases, it is not necessary.

How much your sexual performance will be affected depends on many things and varies from individual to individual. Some people resume their sexual lives shortly after transplant, but for some people it takes months to recover. In those who take longer to recover, sexual performance may be affected by changes in body image, hormonal changes, general level of energy, and physical appearance. Some people make adjustments to their sexual style and focus on intimate times rather than the sexual act itself. If your sexual drive post transplant is reduced, it is important to explore other ways of expressing intimacy such as touching, holding hands, hugging, and kissing. It is essential for you to communicate with your partner openly about your feelings, limitations, desires, and needs. You may start your sexual activity by just having a "touching" session, before you resume normal sexual activity. If you keep having problems, you may want to speak with your doctor about the possibility of hormone replacement therapy.

Communicate with your partner openly about your feelings.

96. Do women have specific problems related to their sexuality post transplant?

Early menopause may frequently affect a woman's sexual drive post transplant. The symptoms of early menopause include hot flashes, vaginal dryness, vaginal tightness, mood shifts, and irritability. Not all women become menopausal, and some women even have children after transplant, although it is rare. For women who do experience early menopause, hormone replacement therapy is an option and may relieve many symptoms such as osteoporosis (weakening of the bones) and coronary heart disease. This is not an option for women with breast cancer, because hormone therapy may increase their chance of relapsing. Women who have vaginal dryness post transplant may use an estrogen cream that they apply directly to their vagina.

97. Will there be changes in my relationships with other people, particularly my family?

The transplant process is very intense and recovery may be prolonged. This process often affects relationships and family ties. In most cases this process brings family members closer; however, sometimes the changes that occur make current tensions worse and cause additional stress. The best way to cope with this is to seek counseling. Open conversations, an attitude of mutual support and understanding, commitment, and spending extra time with affected family members can make a big difference in the outcome of this life-changing situation.

Sometimes the changes that occur make current tensions worse and cause additional stress.

98. Will I have changes in self-esteem post transplant?

Transplant is a very long and difficult experience, and making it through your transplant is quite an accomplishment. However, many things will change after your transplant, such as your physical appearance, physical performance, sexual drive, endurance, and fertility. It is important for you to adjust to these changes and gain a proper understanding of what has happened. As you begin to recover, set realistic goals for yourself and try to achieve them. Do not compare your activity level to that of your healthy friends or colleagues. Do not berate yourself if you are unable to maintain your pre-transplant level of activity. Accept the changes and try to find a new, perhaps even more fulfilling, way of life.

Set realistic goals for yourself.

99. Will I be able to go back to work?

You will not be able to go back to school or work for about 3 to 6 months after an autologous transplant and 7 to 12 months after an allogeneic transplant. How much time you will need to take off from work will depend on what kind of work you do. If you work at home, you may return to work earlier. If your work requires strenuous physical activity, it may take longer before you can return to work. It may also take longer for you to return to work if you work with small children. It is important for you to allow time for a full recovery post transplant so that your immune system is functioning fully before you go back to work. You should consult your physician about this.

Allow time for a full recovery post transplant.

100. Where can I get more information about bone marrow and stem cell transplantation?

This book cannot answer all the questions you might have, so we have compiled a set of resources that will enable you to continue to find answers. The Appendix that follows contains a number of organizations, web sites, books, and other resources that are good sources of reliable information.

Organizations

American Academy of Medical Acupuncture (AAMA)
4929 Wilshire Boulevard, Suite 428
Los Angeles, CA 90010
Phone: 323–937–5514
Web site: *www.medicalacupuncture.org*

American Cancer Society
American Cancer Society National Home Office
1599 Clifton Road
Atlanta, GA 30329
Phone: 800-ACS–2345
Web site: *www.cancer.org*

Blood and Marrow Transplant Information Network
2900 Skokie Valley Rd, Suite B
Highland Park, IL 60035
Phone: 889–597–7674 or 847–433–3313
Web site: *www.bmtinfonet.org*

The Bone Marrow Foundation
70 East 55th Street, 20th floor
New York, NY 10022
Phone: 800–365–1336
Web site: *www.bonemarrow.org*

Cancer Care, Inc.
275 7th Avenue
New York, NY 10001
Phone: 212–712–8400 (administration); 212–712–8080 (services)
Web site: *www.cancercare.org*

Cancer Research Institute
681 Fifth Avenue
New York, NY 10022
Phone: 800–99-CANCER (800–992–26237)
Web site: *www.cancerresearch.org*

Centers for Disease Control and Prevention (CDC)
1600 Clifton Road
Atlanta, GA 30333
Phone: 404–639–3534
800–311–3435
Web site: *www.cdc.gov*

Cure for Lymphoma Foundation
215 Lexington Ave, 11th Floor
New York, NY 10016
Phone: 800–235–6848 or 212–213–9595
Web site: *www.cfl.org*

Department of Veterans Affairs
Veterans Health Association
810 Vermont Avenue, NW
Washington, DC 20420
Phone: 202–273–5400 (Washington, DC office)
800–827–1000 (local VA office)
Web site: *www.va.gov*

Health Insurance Association of America (HIAA)
555 13th Street NW, Suite 600
East Washington, DC 20004–1109
Phone: 202–824–1600
Web site: *www.hiaa.org*

Health Resources and Services Administration
Hill-Burton Program
U.S. Department of Health and Human Services, Parklawn Building
5600 Fishers Lane
Rockville, MD 20857
Phone: 301–443–5656
800–638–0742/800–492–0359 (if calling from the Maryland area)
Web site: *www.hrsa.gov/osp/dfcr/about/aboutdiv.htm*

International Bone Marrow Transplant Registry (IBMTR)
Medical College of Wisconsin
P.O. Box 26509
Milwaukee, WI 53226
Phone: 414 456–8325
Web site: *www.ibmtr.org*

International Cancer Alliance (ICARE)
4853 Cordell Avenue, Suite 11
Bethesda, MD 20814
Phone: 800-ICARE–61 or 301–654–7933
(fax) 201–654–8684
Web site: *www.icare.org/icare*

Leukemia & Lymphoma Society of America
Phone: 800–955–4572 for local chapter information
Web site: *www.leukemia-lymphoma.org*

National Cancer Institute
National Cancer Institute Public Information Office
Building 31, Room 10A31
31 Center Drive, MSC 2580
Bethesda, MD 20892–2580
Phone: 301–435–3848 (public information office line)
Web site: *www.nci.nih.gov*

National Center for Complementary and Alternative Medicine
NCCAM Clearinghouse
P.O. Box 7923
Gaithersburg, MD 20898
Phone: 888–644–6226
Web site: *www.nccam.nih.gov*

National Comprehensive Cancer Network
50 Huntingdon Pike, Suite 200
Rockledge, PA 19046
Phone: 888–909-NCCN (888–909–6226)
Web site: *www.nccn.org*

National Leukemia Research Associations
AKA National Leukemia Research Assn.
585 Stewart Avenue Suite 18
Garden City, NY 11530
Phone: 516–222–1944
Fax: 516–222–0457
Web site: *www.childrensleukemia.org*
NOTE: Although it states only "children's leukemia", there is information on adult leukemia too.

National Marrow Donor Program (NMDP)
3001 Broadway Street NE, Suite 500
Minneapolis, MN 55413
Phone: 800–654–1247 or 612–627–5800
Office of Patient Advocacy
Phone: 888–999–6743
Web site: *www.marrow.org*

Oncology Nursing Society
501 Holiday Drive
Pittsburgh, PA 15220
Phone: 412–921–7373
Web site: *www.ons.org*

Social Security Administration
Office of Public Inquiries
Social Security Administration
Office of Public Inquiries
6401 Security Boulevard, Room 4-C–5 Annex
Baltimore, MD 21235–6401
Phone: 800–772–1213 /800–325–0778 (TTY)
Web site: *www.ssa.gov*

United Seniors Health Cooperative (USHC)
USHC, Suite 200
409 Third Street, SW
Washington, DC 20024
Phone: 202–479–6973
800–637–2604
Web site: *www.unitedseniorshealth.org*

US TOO International, Inc.
903 North York Road, Suite 50
Hinsdale, IL 60521–2993
Phone: 800–808–7866, 630–323–1002
Fax: 630–323–1003
Web site: *www.ustoo.com*

Web Sites with General Cancer Information

Association of Cancer Online Resources, Inc: *www.acor.org*
411Cancer.com
CancerLinks.org
CancerSource.com
CancerWise™/MD Anderson Cancer Center: *www.cancerwise.org*
National Cancer Institute's CancerNet Service: *www.cancernet.nci.nih.gov/index.html.*
Cancerfacts.com
Cancer Supportive Care: *www.cancersupportivecare.com*
Colon Cancer Alliance: *www.ccalliance.org*
Memorial Sloan Kettering Cancer Center: *www.MSKCC.org*

Web Sites with Bone Marrow Transplant Information

www.acor.org
www.bmtinfonet.org
www.cancerbacup.org.uk
www.comnet.org

Web Pages on Specific Topics

Alternative Therapy
Information on acupuncture:
www.medicalacupuncture.org (see American Academy for Medical Acupuncture)

Comprehensive website about alternative therapies for cancer: *www.healthy.net/asp/templates/center.asp?centerid=23*

Chemotherapy

www.yana.org offers online and in person support groups for those going through high dose chemotherapy

Drug information for chemotherapy and hormonal therapy, including information on financial assistance: *www.cancersupportivecare.com/pharmacy.html.*

Clinical Trials

National Cancer Institute's CancerTrials site lists current clinical trials that have been reviewed by NCI. *www.cancertrials.nci.nih.gov*

Coping

National Coalition for Cancer Survivorship (*www.cansearch.org*, 1–877-NCCS-YES) offers a free audio program—"Cancer Survivor Toolbox"—including ways to cope with the illness. Web site also has a newsletter, requiring yearly membership fee.

R. A. Bloch Cancer Foundation (*www.blochcancer.org*) offers an inspirational online book about cancer, relaxation techniques and positive outlooks on fighting cancer, as well as trained one-on-one support from fellow cancer patients.

Diet and Nutrition (Cancer Prevention)

USDA Dietary Guidelines: *www.usda.gov/cnpp*

American Institute for Cancer Research provides tips on how to reduce cancer risk: *www.aicr.org*

Cancer Research Foundation of America's Healthy Eating Suggestions: *www.preventcancer.org/whdiet.cfm*

Family Resources

www.kidscope.org is a website designed to help children understand and cope with the effects of cancer on a parent.

Genetic Counseling

The National Society of Genetic Counselors web site (*www.nsgc.org*) lists society members, complete with specialty.

The National Cancer Institute has a searchable list of health care professionals who specialize in genetics and can provide information and counseling: *cancernet.nci.nih.gov/genesrch.shtml*

Articles on genetics and cancer: *cancer.med.upenn.edu/causeprevent/genetics*

Legal Protections, Financial Resources, and Insurance Coverage

The American Cancer Society offers a number of relevant documents to help understand your coverage and legal protections, and how to find financial assistance. Search *www.cancer.org* using keyword "insurance."

Medicaid Information: *www.hcfa.gov/medical/medicaid.htm*

"Every Question You Need to Ask Before Selling Your Life Insurance Policy." *www.nvrnvr.com*

Family and Medical Leave Act: *www.dol.gov/dol/esa/public/regs/statutes/whd/fmla.htm*

Health Care Financing Administration's (HCFA) information website about Breast Cancer and Medicaid programs: *www.hcfa.gov/medicaid/bccpt/default.htm*

www.needymeds.com offers information about programs sponsored by pharmaceutical manufacturers to help people who cannot afford to purchase necessary drugs.

www.cancercare.org/hhrd/hhrd_financial.htm offers listings of where to look for financial assistance.

The National Financial Resource Book for Patients: A State-by-State Directory: *www.data.patientadvocate.org*

Nausea/Vomiting

National Comprehensive Cancer Network: *www.nccn.org/patient_guidelines/nausea-and-vomiting/nausea-and-vomiting/1_introduction.htm*

Royal Marsden Hospital Patient Information On Line: *www.royalmarsden.org/patientinfo/booklets/coping/nausea7.asp#heading*

Treatment Locators: Physicians and Hospitals

AIM DocFinder (State Medical Board Executive Directors): *www.docboard.org*

Nonprofit organization providing a health professional licensing database.

AMA Physician Select (American Medical Association):
www.ama-assn.org/aps/amahg.htm

AMA database of demographic and professional information on individual physicians in the United States.

American Board of Medical Specialties provides verification of physician qualifications and has lists of specialists. *www.abms.org*, 1–866-ASK-ABMS, or American Board of Medical Specialties, 1007 Church Street, Suite 404, Evanston, IL 60201–5913

Best Hospitals Finder (U.S. News & World Report): *www.usnews.com/usnews/nycu/health/hosptl/tophosp.htm*

The U.S. News hospital rankings are designed to assist patients in their search for the highest level of medical care. Database is searchable by specialty, including the top cancer hospitals (*www.usnews.com/usnews/nycu/health/hosptl/speccanc.htm*) or by geographic region.

Hospital Select (American Medical Association & Medical-Net, Inc.): *www.hospitalselect.com/curb_db/owa/sp_hospselect.main*

Hospital locator database searchable by hospital name, city, state, or zip code. Hospital Select data include basic information (name, address, telephone number), beds and utilization, service lines, and accreditation.

HospitalWeb (Dept. of Neurology, Massachusetts General Hospital):
neuro-www.mgh.harvard.edu/hospitalweb.shtml

Searchable database of hospital web sites.

National Cancer Institute Designated Cancer Centers: *cancertrials.nci.nih.gov/finding/centers/html/map.html*

Directory of NCI-designated Cancer Centers, 58 research-oriented U.S. institutions recognized for scientific excellence and extensive cancer resources. Listings feature phone contact numbers, web site links, and a brief summary of web site resources.

National Comprehensive Cancer Network (NCCN):
www.nccn.org
The National Comprehensive Cancer Network (NCCN) is an alliance of leading cancer centers. NCCN members (*www.nccn.org/profiles.htm*) provide the highest quality in cancer care and cancer research. NCCN offers a patient information and referral service (*www.nccn.org/newsletters/1999_may/page_5.htm*) that responds to cancer-related inquiries and provides referrals to member institutions' programs and services (1–888–909–6226).

Approved Hospital Cancer Program (Commission on Cancer of the American College of Surgeons):
www.facs.org/public_info/yourhealth/aahcp.html
The Approvals Program of the Commission on Cancer surveys hospitals, treatment centers, and other facilities according to standards set by the Committee on Approvals, which recommends approval awards in specific categories based on these surveys. A hospital that has received approval has voluntarily committed itself to providing the best in diagnosis and treatment of cancer. Approved hospitals can be searched by city, state, and category.

Association of Community Cancer Centers: Cancer Centers and Member Profiles:
www.accc-cancer.org/members/map.html
Geographic listing of ACCC members with contact information and description of cancer program and services as provided by the member institutions.

HMOs and Other Managed Care Plans (Cancer Care):
www.cancercare.org/patients/hmos.htm
Discusses the advantages and disadvantages of HMO care.

Physician Qualifications

The American Board of Medical Specialities:
www.abms.org; click on "who's certified" button (search by physician name or by specialty).

Radiation Therapy

National Cancer Institute/CancerNet: Radiation Therapy and You: A Guide to Self-Help During Cancer Treatment. *www.cancernet.nci.nih.gov/peb/radiation/*. By phone, free of charge: 800–4-CANCER (in English and Spanish)

Books and Pamphlets

The following pamphlets are available from the National Cancer Institute by calling 800–4-CANCER:

- "Chemotherapy and You: A Guide to Self-Help During Treatment"
- "Eating Hints for Cancer Patients Before, During, and After Treatment"
- "Get Relief From Cancer Pain"
- "Helping Yourself During Chemotherapy"
- "Questions and Answers About Pain Control: A Guide for People with Cancer and Their Families"
- "Taking Time: Support for People With Cancer and the People Who Care About Them"
- "Taking Part in Clinical Trials: What Cancer Patients Need to Know"

Available in Spanish:

- "Datos sobre el tratamiento de quimioterapia contra el cancer"
- "El tratamiento de radioterapia; guia para el paciente durante el tratamiento"
- "En que consisten los estudios clinicos? Un folleto para los pacientes de cancer"

The following pamphlets are available from the National Comprehensive Cancer Network:

- "Cancer Pain Treatment Guidelines for Patients"
- "Nausea and Vomiting Treatment Guidelines for Patient with Cancer"

Available in Spanish:

- "El dolor asociado con el cáncer"

Carney KL. *What is Cancer Anyway? Explaining Cancer to Children of All Ages*. 1998.

Hapham WH. *When a Parent Has Cancer: A Guide to Caring for Your Children*. 1997.

Landay D. *Be Prepared: The Complete Financial, Legal, and Practical Guide for Living with a Life-challenging Condition.* 1998.

Web Sites and Chat Rooms

cancer.about.com/cs/cancerchatrooms
Memorial Sloan Kettering Cancer Center, *www.mskcc.org*
MD Anderson Cancer Center, *www.mdanderson.org*
Harvard Center for Cancer Prevention, *www.hsph.harvard.edu/cancer*
Cancer Research Foundation of America, *www.crfa.org*

Glossary

ALL: Acute lymphocytic leukemia.

Albumin: A protein produced in the liver that is released into the bloodstream.

Allogeneic stem cell transplantation: Transplant using cells from another person to treat a cancer.

Alopecia: Hair loss resulting from chemotherapy.

Anesthesia: Medication that causes loss of some or all feeling or sensation.

Antiemetic: Medicine that prevents or relieves nausea and vomiting, used during and sometimes after chemotherapy.

Apheresis: Collection of having peripheral blood stem cells.

Aspirate: Removing fluid or cells by inserting a needle into tissue and drawing the fluid into the syringe.

Autologous transplantation: Transplantation using cells from the patient's own body.

Blood count: A test that measures the number of red blood cells (RBCs), white blood cells (WBCs), and platelets in a blood sample.

Blood transfusion: Replenishment of red blood cells in the bloodstream.

Bone marrow: The soft, fatty substance filling the cavities of the bones where blood cells are made.

Bone marrow aspiration biopsy: A procedure in which a needle is inserted into the center of a bone, usually the hip, to remove a small amount of bone marrow for microscopic examination.

Bone marrow harvest: Collection of stem cells from marrow for later infusion into the patient.

Bone marrow transplant (BMT): Transplantation of stem cells collected from bone marrow.

Bulk: Amount of disease.

Cancer: A general term that describes over 100 different uncontrolled growths of abnormal cells in the body. Cancer cells have the ability to continue to grow, invade, and destroy surrounding tissue.

Cancer cell: A cell that divides and reproduces abnormally with uncontrolled growth.

Carcinogen: Any substance that initiates or promotes the development of cancer.

Caregiver: A person who acts for the benefit of a patient at the time of serious illness or disease, on the patient's behalf, and who assists the patient in making decisions and choices.

Catheter, indwelling: Device placed surgically beneath the skin to facilitate the frequent infusion of medications and/or other treatments (see "Port-A-Cath").

Cell: The basic structural unit of all life. All living matter is composed of at least one cell.

Chemotherapy: Treatment of cancer by use of chemicals, and often uses two or more chemicals to achieve maximum kill of tumor cells. Usually refers to drugs used to treat cancer.

Chimerism: The presence of both patient and donor cells together in the bone marrow.

Chromosomes: Large, complex structures that contain DNA and proteins.

Clinical trial: Participating in a designated, specific cancer protocol that has proven to be effective after experiments.

CML: Chronic myeloid leukemia.

CMV: Cytomegalovirus, a virus similar to herpes virus, which can cause pneumonia, hepatitis, and gastrointestinal illness.

COBRA: A legal guarantee of continuation of health coverage offered by insurance companies.

Complete Blood Count (CBC): A laboratory test to determine the number of red blood cells, white blood cells, platelets, hemoglobin and other components of a blood sample.

Conditioning regimen: Chemotherapy designed to prepare for transplant by suppressing the immune system and killing cancer cells.

Consolidation: Additional chemotherapy given in cycles after the initial induction chemotherapy.

Cord blood: Blood retrieved from the umbilical cord of a newborn baby.

Cytotoxic: Drugs that can kill cancer cells. Usually refers to drugs used in chemotherapy treatments.

Diagnosis: The process of identifying a disease by its characteristic signs, symptoms, and laboratory findings.

Discharge planning: The process of preparing a transplant patient to leave the hospital into a controlled, clean, safe environment where the patient has less likelihood of getting an infection post transplant.

DNA: One of two nucleic acids (the other is RNA) found in the nucleus of all cells. DNA contains genetic information on cell growth, division and cell function.

Donor: One who donates blood stem cells or bone marrow for infusion into a patient.

Durable power of attorney for health care: A legal document that allows a patient to name another individual as his or her designated healthcare decision-maker should the patient become too ill to make his or her own decisions in regard to health care.

Engraftment: The process by which a transplant patient's body accepts the donor's cells and incorporates them into normal bodily functions.

Flow cytometry: A test done on cancerous tissues that shows the aggressiveness of the tumor.

Fractionated treatment: See Hyperfractionation.

Full donor chimera: Transformation of a patient's bone marrow to match the bone marrow of his or her donor.

Genes: Located in the nucleus of the cell, genes contain hereditary information that is transferred from cell to cell.

Genetic: Refers to the inherited pattern located in genes for certain characteristics.

Graft-versus-host disease (GVHD): A situation where the lymphocytes from a donor's stem cells recognize certain antigens on the recipient (patient) as foreign.

Graft failure: Rejection of transplanted cells by the recipient.

Graft rejection: See Graft failure.

Granulocyte colony-stimulating-factor (G-CSF): Growth factors given to activate production of cells. A second, related growth factor, **granulocyte-macrophage colony-stimulating-factor (GM-CSF)** may also be given for the same purpose.

Growth factors: Proteins that encourage blood cells to reproduce more rapidly. These are generally used to restore white blood cell counts following treatment.

Hematologist: A specialist who sees and treats patients with malignancies (and other diseases) of the blood.

Hematopoietic stem cell transplant: The process by which new stem cells are introduced into a patient.

Hemolytic anemia: A condition arising when a patient's red blood cells are destroyed by the donor's lymphocytes.

HLA: See Human leukocyte antigen.

HLA-matched sibling: Compatible sister or brother who is determined by testing to be matched at specific loci.

HLA typing: Tests to determine the antigens present in a person's cells.

Human leukocyte antigen: Antigens that act as markers on each person's cells that help the body distinguish its own cells from invading or foreign cells.

Hyperfractionation: A dose of radiation given in several sessions instead of all at once. Also called **fractionated treatment**.

Immune system: Complex system by which the body protects itself from outside invaders that are harmful to it.

Immunocompromised: A condition in which a patient's immune system is unable to perform its functions adequately, leaving the patient vulnerable to infections.

Immunotherapy: Treatment that stimulates the body's own defense mechanisms to combat diseases such as cancer.

Immunosuppressed: Condition of having a lowered resistance to disease. May be a temporary result of lowered white blood cell counts from chemotherapy administration.

Induction therapy: Chemotherapy that suppresses the patient's immune system prior to transplantation.

Informed consent: A process in which all risks and complications of a procedure or treatment are explained to a patient before the procedure is done. Most informed consents are written and signed by the patient or a legal representative.

Intravenous (IV): entering the body through a vein.

Leukemia: A malignancy of a white blood cell in which there is an abnormal accumulation of white blood cells in the blood and the bone marrow.

Leukocyte: A white blood cell or corpuscle.

Lymphocyte: Leukocytes made in lymphoid tissue that are typical cellular elements of lymph, and include cellular mediators of immunity, constituting 20–30% of leukocytes of normal human blood.

Malaise: A condition marked by fatigue and overall poor feeling.

Matched sibling transplant (MST): A transplant in which the stem cells come from a relative, usually a sibling, in whom all six of the six HLA antigens are identical to the patient's HLA antigens.

Matched unrelated donor (MUD) transplant: A transplant in which the stem cells are obtained from an unrelated donor whose HLA antigens match at least some of the patient's. A MUD transplant has a lower chance of success than a MST transplant.

Microorganism: An organism of minute, microscopic size.

Molecular remission: When special tests that amplify small numbers of cells can determine whether the disease is totally eradicated.

Mucositis: A temporary but painful condition where the lining of the inside of the mouth breaks down, making eating and swallowing difficult.

Mulipotent stem cell: A stem cell that can form many kinds of the same bodily tissue, e.g., a hematopoietic stem cell is one that can form all different types of blood cells.

Multipotent stem cell: A stem cell that can form many different kinds of body tissues.

NMDP: National Marrow Donor Program: A large registry with millions of potential donors in its files.

Neutropenic diet: A diet used by people with suppressed immune systems that limits intake of fresh foods in order to lower the possibility of infection.

Neutropenia: A condition in which the body is depleted of important disease-fighting white blood cells.

Neutrophil: A common type of white blood cell.

Nonmyeloablative stem cell transplant (NST): An allogeneic transplant with less toxicity in which only part of the patient's bone marrow is destroyed by chemotherapy before the transplant. Donor cells then kill the patient's cancer cells.

Oncologist: A physician who specializes in cancer treatment.

Oncology: The science dealing with the physical, chemical, and biological properties and features of cancer, including causes, the disease process, and therapies.

Parenteral nutrition: Nutrition supplied intravenously instead of by mouth.

Patient advocate: An individual who serves the needs of the patient, who may be empowered to act on his/her behalf.

PBSC: *See* Peripheral blood stem cell.

Peripheral blood: Blood that passes through the arteries and veins to supply oxygen to the tissues and organs.

Peripheral blood stem cell: Stem cells that are circulating freely within the blood and can be collected through apheresis. Most stem cells are found in bone marrow, but can be encouraged to move into the peripheral blood for collection.

Pharmaceuticals: Medications that are continuously being developed for future patient care.

Platelet: A cell formed by the bone marrow and circulating in the blood that is necessary for blood clotting.

Port-A-Cath: A catheter device surgically implanted under the skin, usually on the chest, that enters a large blood vessel and is used to deliver medication, chemotherapy, and blood products, and also is used to obtain blood samples.

Preparative regimen: *See* Conditioning regimen.

Pre-transplant work up: The series of tests and evaluations of the patient's physical condition that determine whether the patient is capable of handling a transplant.

Prognosis: A prediction of the course of the disease—the future prospects for the patient's life and welfare.

Protocol: A regimen of selected drugs and treatment time intervals known to be effective against a certain cancer.

Purge: To clean out or remove diseased cells from tissue, in this case bone marrow.

Radiation therapy: Treatment with high energy x-rays to destroy cancer cells.

Relapse: The reappearance of cancer after a disease-free period.

Red blood cells: Hemoglobin-containing blood cells that carry oxygen to the tissues.

Remission: Complete or partial disappearance of the signs and symptoms of disease in response to treatment; the period during which a disease is under control.

Risk factors: Anything that increases an individual's chance of getting a disease such as cancer.

Secondary cancers: A second site where cancer is found.

Side effects: Effects of treatment other than the desired effects. This usually describes situations that occur after treatments. For example, hair loss may be a side effect of chemotherapy, and fatigue may be a side effect of radiation therapy.

Stem cell: A primitive type of cell from which all cells of a given organ or tissue arise.

Stem cell transplant: The process by which new stem cells are infused into a patient.

Surface marker: A protein on the surface of a cell that helps identify the cell.

Syngeneic transplant: A transplant from an identical twin.

TBI: *See* Total body irradiation.

T-cell depleted transplant: A transplant in which lymphocytes are removed from the donated bone marrow prior to transplantation.

Total body irradiation: Radiation therapy given over the whole body to remove all cancer or disease cells and suppress the immune system; TBI dose is precisely calculated by the radiation oncologist to remove all indication of disease.

Totipotent stem cell: A stem cell that can form any type of tissue in the body.

Tissue: A collection of similar cells. There are four basic types of tissues in the body: epithelial, connective, muscle, and nerve.

Tumor: An abnormal tissue, swelling, or mass; may be either benign or malignant.

Translocation: The movement of one piece of chromosome to another chromosome.

Vaso-occlusive disease (VOD): A sometimes fatal condition that can lead to liver failure; requires rapid medical intervention.

White blood cells: A blood cell that does not contain hemoglobin; also called leukocytes. White blood cells fight disease and heal injuries.

Index

U

V

W

Z

Notes

Notes

Notes

Notes

Notes

Notes